CANCER

If curable, why not cured?

CANCER

If curable, why not cured?

BY

J. S. MITCHELL

C.B.E., F.R.S.

Regius Professor of Physic in the University of Cambridge, and Fellow of St John's College

W. HEFFER AND SONS LTD

CAMBRIDGE

1971

Published by
W. HEFFER AND SONS LTD
20 Trinity Street, Cambridge, England

ISBN 0 85270 050 4

Printed in Great Britain by W. Heffer and Sons Ltd

To the Master
Fellows and Scholars of
St John's College
Cambridge

Arrangements have been made for royalties from the sale of this book to be paid into Professor Mitchell's Research Fund, University of Cambridge.

CONTENTS

PREFACE

This book is an expanded version of the Linacre Lecture, which I delivered in Cambridge on 6 May 1970. While preserving the essential features of the lecture, it includes in addition the details of the evidence, which are necessary for a critical appraisal of the medical, scientific and administrative problems discussed.

The book expresses an essentially personal view. I hope that it may be of interest to those concerned with the care, diagnosis and treatment of patients with cancer and to those involved in research and development in this field. I have always thought it is most desirable to encourage a close association between the practical clinical and research aspects of this subject. In my own Department in Cambridge, the policy of having the clinic and at least some of the research laboratories close together in the same building has been very helpful to the patients and has often stimulated new ideas in research and development.

At the present time, the most important factor limiting the diagnosis and treatment of patients with cancer appears to be lack of knowledge. There is an urgent need for much more clinical and laboratory research in relation to the problem of cancer, not only what is now called 'mission-oriented' research but also fundamental and 'curiosity-based' research. The stimulation of fundamental research to the best advantage is one of the problems of our time. An important question is whether we can apply the results of fundamental science to the diagnosis and treatment of patients with cancer more rapidly today than in the past.

Finally, may I say that, although we are likely to be influenced to an ever-increasing extent by scientific methods and the results of scientific research, we must never forget the human side of the treatment of the patient.

JOSEPH S. MITCHELL

ADDENBROOKE'S HOSPITAL
CAMBRIDGE

6 July 1970

ACKNOWLEDGEMENTS

First, I wish to acknowledge my gratitude to my wife, Dr L. Mary Mitchell, not only for her advice about the preparation of the Linacre Lecture and of this book but also for her continued help in the course of the work upon which it is based and for her expert medical supervision of the records of the Radiotherapeutic Centre, Addenbrooke's Hospital.

I wish to take this opportunity of acknowledging the help and encouragement I have received from my colleagues on the staff of Addenbrooke's Hospital, of the Radiotherapeutic Centre and of the Department of Radiotherapeutics, University of Cambridge. I wish to thank them all. In addition, I acknowledge the great help I have received from Mr E. A. King and for his skilled assistance in the animal experiments. I thank Mr. E. W. Mitchell for the preparation of a number of the photographs.

I wish to thank my secretary, Miss Mary J. Crichton, for her great help and patience in the preparation of the manuscript. I am particularly indebted to Mrs G. R. Cant for preparing the index of Subjects and Authors.

I wish to thank the Editors of the following publications for permission to include illustrations: *Acta Radiologica* for Fig. 3 and the loan of blocks; *Strahlentherapie* for Fig. 5; *Strahlenschäden-Strahlenschutz* for Fig. 6.

I would like to express my thanks to Messrs W. Heffer and Sons Ltd for their helpfulness in the publication of this book.

Last, but not least, the publication of this book was assisted by a donation in memory of the late Mrs Nora Burns of Cambridge.

I

Introduction

The Linacre Lectureship in Physic at St John's College, Cambridge, was founded in 1524 by Thomas Linacre but it never played an important part in medical education in the University. In 1908 the Lectureship was revived and the first of these annual lectures was given by Sir William Osler. It was devoted perhaps understandably to Linacre himself – seen as medical humanist, physician, grammarian, translator, teacher and last but not least founder and first President of the Royal College of Physicians. I can only feel very humble when I recall the Linacre Lectures I have heard and when I read the list of Lecturers and realise what a great honour and responsibility it is to be invited to be one, particularly by my own College.

Some aspects of cancer have been considered in previous Linacre Lectures. In 1927, Dr J. A. Murray, Director of the Imperial Cancer Research Fund spoke about 'Multiple New Growths'. Two years later, Dr F. Peyton Rous chose as his title 'The Modern Dance of Death'. This was the first Linacre Lecture I heard and I still remember it well. At that time, many people were sceptical about Peyton Rous's work and it was suggested afterwards that the students did not take the lecture too seriously. However, after many years, the importance of his work on viruses as one of the factors that can play a part in causing malignant tumours is now generally recognised.

Traditionally, the Linacre Lecture is an occasion to present a statement of general interest with scientific accuracy. I have chosen my subject because of its importance to all of us as an outstanding medical and scientific problem of our time with major social implications and because it has been the main theme of my own work and that of my colleagues. This lecture is an attempt to take stock of the present position concerning the treatment of people with cancer and to consider new approaches to the problems in some detail. (I shall avoid any unpleasant pictures). It is of course a personal view emphasising my own interests and those of my colleagues in the context of present knowledge of the subject. I would like to take this opportunity of thanking my many colleagues for their help and support over the years.

I shall start with a brief account of some aspects of the efforts which have been made throughout the world to improve the treatment and care of patients with cancer and allied diseases, particularly in the last 25 years and with emphasis on the more recent developments and ideas. I shall try to make an assessment both of the not inconsiderable progress made already and of the serious practical, clinical and scientific problems still to be solved. After the general introduction, I shall select four topics for particular consideration, viz.,

(1) the assessment of the results of treatment and especially of new methods,

(2) some work in progress, of both clinical and scientific interest,

(3) some considerations of the mechanisms of the therapeutic actions of ionising radiations, and

(4) problems of organisation.

First looking briefly to the past, may I say from my own experience how greatly the treatment of patients with cancer and allied diseases has improved since I started as a medical student (in Birmingham) in 1926. At that time, in Europe, North America and Great Britain, the use of radium was becoming an accepted method of treatment, particularly for cancer of the uterine cervix. In this country, the work of the Paris school, especially the clinical and radiobiological studies of Claude Regaud, had a great influence. It was also in 1926 that H. J. Muller made the fundamental discovery that in the fruit fly, Drosophila, X-rays were able to induce mutations indistinguishable from those which appeared spontaneously; it is depressing to note that this remarkable scientific work had extraordinarily little influence on medical radiobiology for many years. In 1928, the 'roentgen' unit for measurement of the dose of X-rays was accepted by international agreement and Gösta Forssell of Stockholm published his book *On the permanency of radiological healing in malignant tumours*. In the U.K., the National Radium Trust and the Radium Commission were established in 1929. This was a time of development, and of enthusiasm which was estimable but which in retrospect was sometimes uncritical. However, the tremendous amount of scientific and clinical information presented in Lazarus' *Handbuch der gesamten Strahlenheilkunde*, in Vol. I, 1928, and Vol. II, 1931, was in striking contrast to the assessment of the position in 1910 as given in the Encyclopaedia Britannica: 'the only "cure" for cancer remains removal by operation; . . . Until more is known both of cancer and of X-rays, their use must be considered not only experimental but risky'. It is useful to emphasise that the advances in this field were largely due to co-ordinated efforts among workers in many disciplines. Particularly important was what Russ called 'the heritage of physics and its application in cancer'.

I think that cancer should be discussed openly and considered as objectively as possible. One must recognise the difficulty that cancer is a subject about which few people, including doctors, can think without emotion. However, slowly with increasing knowledge and education and psychological understanding, together with steadily improving methods of diagnosis, treatment and care, we must try to get over these fears and anxieties. I have found that in recent years many more patients want to know the exact position. However, some do not and some patients who have been told the position, insist that this is not so. I think that while one does one's best to be kind and hopeful, it is in general wise to discuss the position honestly with all those concerned, particularly to avoid barriers between a husband and wife. However, even among intelligent people, there is a deeply ingrained belief that nothing useful can be done. If a patient with cancer does well and at least returns to apparently normal health, people often say 'it could not have been as serious as we had feared'.

A BRIEF INTRODUCTION TO SOME BASIC TOPICS

A useful though over-simplified picture of the process of development of a malignant tumour is that uncontrolled cell division leads to the formation of a tumour mass, which as it develops not only may cause pressure but also often actively invades adjacent structures and at some stage sheds off malignant cells or groups of cells, which spread by the blood stream or lymphatic vessels to form secondary tumours – metastases – at a distance. It may be mentioned here that, as a rule, and contrary to common belief, localised cancer is *not* painful. (In this lecture, I shall often use the term cancer to include all types of malignant neoplasms.) The distinction between malignant and normal cells is not the fact that cancer cells grow. Perhaps the most important feature is that normal cells cease to grow when growth is no longer required, whereas cancer cells multiply with uninhibited proliferation and without regard to the needs and well-being of the organism as a whole. From a biological point of view, the development of cancer appears to be a very complicated process and there is a great deal of evidence which is incompatible with a purely cytological explanation (Smithers, 1962; Burch, 1970). The problem is an extraordinarily difficult one. There is a tremendous amount of evidence available from many fields including molecular biology, general and cell biology, genetics, biochemistry, virology, radiobiology, pathology, immunology, pharmacology, endocrinology, epidemiology, medicine, surgery and gynaecology.

Reference must be made here of the far-reaching concept of the hormonal dependence and responsiveness of certain malignant tumours; this is now a major field of study and is particularly important in the treatment of carcinoma of the prostate and some cases of carcinoma of the breast.

In a possibly related but much less well-investigated field, there are many unsolved problems concerning psychosomatic aspects of malignant disease (Kissen and LeShan, 1964). Not infrequently one observes the recurrence of a malignant tumour which has been healed for many years, after emotional upheaval such as follows the death of a husband, wife or child (Mitchell, 1960). This phenomenon of the clinical manifestation of the recurrence of an apparently healed malignant tumour, within a year and sometimes within a few months, after a bereavement, has been observed by a number of clinicians; however, I think that this is a problem which should be studied critically by means of a prospective clinical trial. I should also like to mention that occasionally patients have what appears to be a subconscious knowledge of the presence of a tumour in a particular organ, e.g. breast, or colon. This is a difficult subject because many people at some time think they may have a cancer, when this turns out not to be the case.

The biochemical effects of the tumour on the host are as yet little understood but are being investigated. In recent years, 'ectopic' hormone production by many non-endocrine tumours has been generally recognised and is of practical clinical importance quite apart from its scientific interest and implications (see Ross, 1968; Goodall, 1969). Similarly, a number of human tumours produce an ectopic alkaline phosphatase isoenzyme, the Regan isoenzyme, indistinguishable from molecular Variant B of placental alkaline phosphatase (Fishman, 1969).

Further, the discovery of characteristic antigens in tumour cells has led to a revival of the study of tumour immunology of major importance and great promise, particularly I think for diagnosis. (See e.g. Harris, 1967). A problem which is still unresolved, is raised by the very rare, though real occurrence, of apparently spontaneous healing of human malignant tumours – in perhaps about 1 in 10,000 cases of all types of tumours in adults.

There is now a great deal of quantitative evidence about the growth of malignant tumours. The size of the primary tumour depends not only on the rate of division of the tumour cells but also on the proportion of non-proliferating tumour cells present, which is often substantial (Mendelsohn, 1960) and perhaps more surprisingly, on the rate of loss of tumour cells, which has been found often to amount to between 90 and 99% of the rate of cell proliferation (Refsum and Berdal, 1967; Steel, 1968; Iversen, 1967; Tubiana, Frindel and Malaise, 1969). In fact, most human malignant tumours grow much more slowly than might be expected. It is reasonable to assume that in a tumour with its connective tissue stroma, there are about 10^8 malignant cells per cm^3. (It is difficult to regard a tumour of volume 1 cc as genuinely early; it is to be noted that a tumour of volume 1 cu mm which would usually be very difficult to detect, contains about 10^5 malignant cells.) A metastasis or a recurrence starting from a single cell, with a volume doubling time of 66 days – which is a typical average value – would take about 5 years to reach a volume of 1 cm^3. The tendency to form metastases varies enormously with different types of tumour and with tumours of apparently the same pathological type in different individuals. However, many tumour cells which are shed off into the blood stream, and probably also into the lymphatics, seem to disappear rapidly and only a very few ultimately develop into clinical metastases. A striking example of this is seen in cases of carcinoma of the uterine cervix both during radical surgery and during radium insertion. (Wimhöfer, Wagner and Schunck, 1963). There can be little doubt that there are host defence mechanisms against both primary and secondary malignant tumours, though it is often difficult to assess their importance. Almost certainly, a component of the defence mechanisms is cellular, involving lymphocytes. It is obviously important to try to develop methods for the prevention of metastases (e.g. Gasic, Gasic and Stewart, 1968) and to study the mechanisms involved by all available methods, including e.g. physicochemical studies of the properties of the surfaces of normal and malignant cells using microelectrophoresis (Ambrose, James and Lowick, 1956; Simon-Reuss, Cook, Seaman and Heard, 1964; Mehrishi, 1969) and biological studies of the penetration of the vascular endothelial barrier by both neoplastic and non-neoplastic cells (Fisher and Fisher, 1967; Taptiklis, 1969).

It is my view that the much discussed problem of the early diagnosis of malignant disease needs to be looked at critically. Early treatment is always advocated and there can be little doubt that from a practical point of view, it is almost invariably wise. However, it must be clearly stated that there is by no means universal agreement that length of delay after the onset of symptoms greatly affects the prognosis. The problems are particularly difficult in cancer of breast, where the degree of malignancy of the tumour, assessed in terms of some form of pathological grading (Bloom, 1950; Cutler *et al.*, 1969) and host response to the tumour (Hamlin, 1968) are of great importance. Nevertheless, in the Registrar General's Statistical Review of England and Wales for the year 1961; Supplement on Cancer (1967) it was shown that in 21,018 cases of cancer of the breast in women as delay before seeking treatment increased, the prognosis deteriorated from a crude 5-year survival rate of 54% in those reporting in the first month to 41% for those with a history of 6 months and 38% in those delaying over 2 years.

This problem must be considered from a biological point of view. The smallest clinically detectable tumour is often perhaps 3 mm in diameter and contains between about one and two million malignant cells. It is obviously desirable to try to find some method of detecting malignant tumours at a much earlier stage. Perhaps immunological methods will prove of value. There is evidence that *presymptomatic treatment* can be valuable, e.g. in the case of carcinoma of the rectum at a Cancer Detection Centre (Gilbertson and Wangensteen, 1964). However, special mention must be made of the well-known use of the cytology of smears to detect precancerous lesions of the uterine cervix – carcinoma *in situ* – and treat these, and also the early invasive carcinomatous lesions discovered at the smear test, without delay (see e.g. McLaren, 1963). This development presents many problems. However, the remarkable studies carried out in the screening programme in British Columbia show that a significant reduction in the incidence of invasive carcinoma of the cervix has been achieved (Fiddler, Boyes and Worth, 1968). In a letter dated 20 April 1970 Dr D. A. Boyes has kindly told me that 'The decline in mortality (for squamous carcinoma of the cervix) is possibly significant, it certainly is statistically but we cannot, of course, be certain that this decline results from our programme'.

THE MAGNITUDE OF THE TASK

Apart from research and development, the magnitude of the task of providing treatment and care for all the individual patients with cancer presents formidable problems. In a number of European countries – with at least 15% of the population over the age of 60 – there are about 3,300 to 3,500 new cases of malignant disease of all types per million of the population per year (see W.H.O., 1966); here in the East Anglian region of England, the figure was 3,374 for the year 1967–68 (see Cancer Records Bureau, 1969). In England and Wales in the year 1968, cancer (all forms) was the second commonest cause of death; it constituted 19·5% of all causes of death, whereas all diseases of the heart and circulatory system accounted for 51% and deaths from motor vehicle accidents 1·1% (Annual Rept. C.M.O., 1969).

The problem of cancer is world-wide (see Doll, Payne and Waterhouse, 1966). It is interesting that the incidence of different types of cancer varies greatly in different parts of the world (Dunham and Bailar, 1968). There is a very high incidence of cancer of the lung in men in the United Kingdom, of cancer of the stomach in men on the U.S.S.R., Japan and Iceland and of cancer of the uterine cervix in women among the Puerto Ricans in New

York City and in Columbia. It is well known that there is a generally low incidence of cancer of the cervix in Jewish women; another relevant finding is the low incidence of cancer of the breast in women in Japan and the U.S.S.R. Mention may also be made of the relatively high incidence of cancer of the mouth and pharynx in India and cancer of the nasopharynx in China, together with cancer of the bladder in Argentina, Mozambique, Egypt and Sudan and cancer of the skin in Australia.

It is a tragic fact that in England and Wales, the death rate from cancer of the lung (which is largely carcinoma of the bronchus and is much more common in men than women) has been increasingly steadily. However, the work of Doll (1967) showed that since 1957 the mortality from cancer of the lung in British male doctors has decreased. Considering the mortality from lung cancer among men aged 35–84 years standardised for age, the death rates per 1,000 per year for British doctors decreased from 1·10 in 1953–57 to 0·83 in 1961–65 and for the male population of England and Wales increased from 1·49 to 1·88 for the same periods (Doll, 1970, personal communication). It is difficult to avoid the conclusion that the decrease in mortality among male doctors is because many stopped smoking cigarettes as soon as the association with lung cancer was publicised.

A DISCUSSION OF METHODS OF TREATMENT

In discussing methods of treatment I want to emphasise the need to consider the patient with cancer as an individual human being. As well as treating the person concerned, we must support the whole family. At the present time, the methods of treatment of cancer, which always have to be considered in reaching a decision about each patient, are (1) first and foremost surgery, (2) radiotherapy and (3) chemotherapy and various combinations of these three methods. Immunological methods are being investigated. The indications in each case depend upon a great many factors. Often the decision as to the best line of action is reached as a result of consultation between a number of specialists; however, it is my view that it is important for one doctor to be finally responsible for the decisions concerning the individual patient. Only rarely does one decide initially to give no active treatment, apart from symptomatic measures. General medical treatment before, during and after treatment is an essential part of the management of the patient. With any form of treatment it is wise to try to avoid impairment of the 'host resistance'.

The emphasis in this lecture is on cure. However, although every effort is made to cure patients with cancer and despite the progress that has been made, it is unfortunately the case that there are and will be many patients who cannot be cured. Almost all of these can be helped tremendously and constructively by palliative treatment and as a result many return to normal health and the enjoyment of life. Relief of pain is essential and is possible to a much greater extent than is commonly believed. May I say that since the work of Dogliotti in 1936, I have been particularly interested in the treatment of otherwise intractable pain by relatively simple procedures of nerve blocking (see e.g. Youngman, 1965). When the end is approaching, a tremendous amount can be done. An impressive approach to the problem of 'terminal care' is the work of Dr Cicely Saunders at St Christopher's Hospice, London. However, many patients die at home. An experienced general practitioner (Wilkes, 1970) estimated that about one in eight cases of cancer dying at home need 'heavy and demanding care' from the doctor for up to six weeks and points out the need 'of a place where hospital standards of nursing care are available to both the relatives and the general practitioner'. I can confirm the reality of this need in many parts of this country, including East Anglia. It is my view that doctors looking after patients with cancer in the last stages, must take responsibility for relieving pain and distress and are not doing their duty unless they do so effectively. I and many doctors I know, do not hesitate to give sufficient drugs when necessary to make the end peaceful. Voluntary euthanasia has had many advocates including Sir Thomas More in his

Utopia (1516). On the basis of my own experience with patients I must express my own personal opinion against its legalisation, though I appreciate only too well what a difficult subject this is. Nevertheless, I felt it must be considered, at least briefly, before discussing the more technical aspects of methods of treatment.

Complete surgical removal of a tumour is obviously likely to cure the patient. However, this is by no means always possible, because microscopic spread of malignant cells may have occurred already. For example, tumour cells can be found in the bone marrow in some otherwise operable cases of carcinoma of the bronchus (Kingsley Pillers, 1955, 1965; Kingsley Pillers, Marks and Mitchell, 1956). Unrecognised spread of the malignant cells is probably the most important single cause of failure to cure the malignant disease; however, in some cases, the malignant cells are present and latent, possibly dormant, for some years perhaps even indefinitely without producing any disease. This type of evidence and the study of host defence mechanisms has contributed to the recent re-appraisal of the place of surgery in malignant disease, with a movement toward more limited operative procedures, particularly, as we shall see, for cancer of the breast.

Radiotherapy is important because apart from surgery, ionizing radiations are the only agents, which as yet have cured large numbers of patients with cancer. However, even when there is no possibility of cure, less intensive radiotherapy, in conjunction with good medical management, is often of great palliative value especially in relieving distressing symptoms, of which pain is by far the most important and not infrequently restores the patient to normal health at least for a time. Useful palliative treatment involves a period, often months, of essentially normal active life and the end when it comes is usually rapid, and not a slow deterioration. In a very small proportion of cases, radiotherapy which was palliative in its intention, proves to be curative.

In the last 25 years, there has been a great practical improvement in radiotherapy, mainly as a result of the use of high energy radiations. This has been made possible by the introduction of radio-cobalt ^{60}Co, produced by nuclear reactors (Dunworth and Mitchell, 1945; Mitchell, 1946) and the subsequent wide availability of gamma-ray teletherapy units, and the development and manufacture of linear accelerators and betatrons, producing X-rays and fast electrons of energies mainly from 4 to 45 MeV (million electron volts). The International Atomic Energy Agency (1968) reported that for use in radiotherapy throughout the world, in 1967 there were 1676 ^{60}Co teletherapy units and 140 ^{137}Cs teletherapy units together with 137 betatrons, 79 linear accelerators, 20 Van de Graaff machines and 7 resonant transformer X-ray generators.

In Cambridge our two ^{60}Co units arrived only in 1962 and 1967; to meet our needs, we developed a 20 Ci ^{192}Ir unit (Freundlich, Haybittle and Quick, 1950) and in 1957 installed a 1700 Ci ^{137}Cs unit designed here (Haybittle and Dallison, 1958) and constructed in the University Engineering Laboratory workshops. We used a synchrotron producing 30 MeV X-rays, provided by the Medical Research Council, for treating patients from 1951 to 1959; the radiation was very useful but was delivered at an inconveniently low dose rate and the machine was unreliable (Mitchell, 1960). Through the good offices of the late Sir John Cockroft, a 15 MeV linear accelerator was made available and we have been treating patients routinely with it since June 1963, using mainly the 15 MeV X-rays but also 14 MeV electrons in some cases.

From the patient's point of view, radiotherapy with high energy radiation is usually much less disturbing and produces far less severe reactions of the skin than with older 'deep X-rays'. With high energy radiations, the scope of radiotherapy has been widened substantially and in general, the techniques of treatment have been improved and often simplified. The use of computers in radiotherapy was first described by Tsien (1955) and has increased the information available in dose calculations and the accuracy of practical treatment planning (see e.g. Mitchell and Sterling, 1967); it can now be regarded as a routine procedure. The use of a multi-access computer for this purpose in Cambridge has been described by Haybittle and Houston (1968). However, caution is necessary in the assessment of the results of radiotherapy with high-energy radiations though there is already some evidence suggesting improvement of the long-term results of treatment in certain types of malignant disease, especially carcinoma of the antrum and of the oropharynx, carcinoma of the cervix, Stage III, carcinoma of the bladder and of seminoma of the testis.

In addition to the use of high energy radiations, there has been a steady improvement of techniques of radiotherapy and of associated diagnostic methods. As an example of this, it is of particular interest that the long-term results in the treatment of Hodgkin's disease have improved tremendously (see e.g. Peters, 1950; Kaplan, 1966; Easson and Russell, 1968; Lacher, 1969; Smithers, 1969). Easson and Russell (1968) of Manchester, report survival rates (age-corrected) at 15 years after initial radiotherapy of 39% in 103 localised cases of Hodgkin's disease and 13% in 216 not-localised cases; moreover, there is every indication that since 1960, the results of treatment of patients with Hodgkin's disease have improved still further (Smithers, 1969).

Thought about radiotherapy has been influenced greatly as a result of the demonstration by Puck, Marcus and Cieciura (1956) of the feasibility of growing single mammalian cells in a manner rather similar to bacterial cells, so that each develops into a visible colony (clone). These cells, both normal and malignant, were found to be extremely radiosensitive. A new field of radiobiology has developed on the basis of this technique. The results have been illuminating from a quantitative point of view but there are still outstanding problems in their application to radiotherapy. Perhaps the most difficult of these is the role of 'host responses'. A great deal of work is in progress, particularly in this country, to try to improve the results of radiotherapy of many types of tumours by the use of hyperbaric oxygen inhaled in a suitable tank at 3 atmospheres pressure before and during irradiation in certain cases – to try to overcome the radioresistance of anoxic cells in tumours – and also by the use of chemical radiosensitizers.

An apparently valuable though unspectacular application of radiobiology in radiotherapy is the use of blood transfusions to maintain a physiological level of haemoglobin during treatment.

At present there is a renewed interest in the therapeutic possibilities of fast neutrons, because they produce greater damage to anoxic cells for the same damage to well-oxygenated cells, than with X-rays, gamma-rays and electrons; a clinical trial of fast neutron therapy has been started at Hammersmith Hospital, London, in conjunction with the Medical Research Council's cyclotron unit (Fowler, 1967; Morgan, 1967, 1968). Consideration should be given to the possibilities of the uses of sealed fast neutron sources of californium-252 (Wright *et al.*, 1967) or of curium-242-beryllium (Radiochemical Centre, Amersham, 1970) for implants or intracavitary application in radiotherapy. There is still a need for critical studies of the dosimetry of fast neutrons (see e.g. Broerse and Barendsen, 1970).

With regard to other radiations, mention must be made of the clinical investigations of neutron capture therapy in the post-operative treatment of patients with glioblastoma multiforme at the nuclear reactor at Brookhaven (Farr, Sweet *et al.*, 1954); this method was based on the capture of slow neutrons by the boron isotope, ^{10}B, with disintegration and release of the densely ionizing particles of ^{4}He and ^{7}Li in the tumour tissue where there was some selective concentration of borate after intravenous injection. The therapeutic possibilities of various heavy particles of high energy, viz. protons, deuterons, α-particles and the heavy ions of carbon, oxygen, neon and argon have been examined; biological experiments have been started with negative pi-mesons. (Fowler and Perkins, 1961; see also Lawrence and Tobias, 1967). Kjellberg *et al.* (1962) reported on the use of 160 MeV protons from the Harvard cyclotron for Bragg peak irradiation of patients with cerebral tumours and 185 MeV protons have been used for radiotherapy 'on a moderate scale' at Uppsala. (Falkmer, Fors and Larsson, 1962; Graffman and Jung, 1970.) It is to be noted that these high energy protons do not differ appreciably in their biological effects from other low LET radiations such as ^{60}Co γ-rays and accordingly do not share the potential capacity of fast neutrons, negative pions and heavy nuclei for damaging anoxic tumour cells.

Developments of this type are extremely costly and attention has turned to the possibilities of simple methods of improving the techniques of radiotherapy. In recent years, there has been a revival of interest in the problem of dose fractionation, particularly from the radiobiological point of view (see e.g. Strandqvist, 1963; Ellis, 1967; Mitchell and Mitchell, 1967; Cohen and Scott, 1968; Sambrook, 1968; Hall, 1969). Moreover, irradiation at low dose rates for long periods will probably reduce the Oxygen Enhancement Ratio (Hall, Bedford and Oliver, 1966) and also be associated with increased re-oxygenation of surviving anoxic tumour cells (Maeda and Suit, 1965; Thomlinson, 1966; van Putten, 1968; van Putten and Kallmann, 1968). Both these effects are likely to reduce the radioresistance of tumours. It is my view that they are particularly relevant to the development of long-term implants and of radioactive drugs.

Turning to the therapeutic uses of radio-isotopes, it is of interest that in recent years, radium is being replaced by equivalent sources of radio-caesium-137 of half-life 30 years, in tubes for use in suitable applicators in the treatment of carcinoma of the cervix, and in needles for interstitial therapy, mainly because of the greater safety in handling and ease of protection of the staff. Radon seeds have been replaced by radio-gold-198 'grains'. A number of other isotopes have also been used, e.g. ^{90}Y rods for pituitary ablation in certain advanced cases of cancer of the breast and ^{182}Ta and ^{192}Ir wire for interstitial small volume irradiation in carcinoma of the bladder and various tumours of the brain (Mundinger, 1969). Mention must also be made of intralymphatic therapy, with lipiodol incorporating ^{131}I, as iodinated triolein, or ^{32}P as tri-n-octyl phosphate and the uses of radioactive colloids, particularly radioactive colloidal gold, ^{198}Au, colloidal chromic phosphate ^{32}P, and colloidal yttrium silicate – ^{90}Y, and of suspensions of ceramic microspheres containing ^{90}Y (see e.g. Müller, 1961; Jantet, 1969). The external use of isotopes emitting high energy β-rays, especially ^{90}Sr, has been found of practical value in ophthalmic applicators for the treatment of both non-malignant and malignant conditions of the eye (Lederman 1953, 1956) and in the multicurie teletherapy sources developed in Cambridge. In 1960, Dr J. L. Haybittle described a 10 Ci ^{90}Sr β-ray therapy unit. This was subsequently improved to include a moving couch technique (Horwitz and Haybittle, 1960). Then Dr Haybittle (1964) developed a moving 24 Ci ^{90}Sr unit for whole-body superficial irradiation with β-rays. Since then, my colleagues, especially Dr D. G. Bratherton, and I have found this apparatus is extremely useful in the treatment of patients with widespread superficial skin diseases, especially the rare but very unpleasant condition, mycosis fungoides.

In medical treatment, the internal administration of radio-isotopes is of great practical value in a few limited fields, mainly the use of the radio-iodine, ^{131}I, in selected cases of thyrotoxicosis and certain cases of carcinoma of the thyroid and to a lesser extent, the use of radiophosphorus, ^{32}P, in polycythaemia vera. These radio-isotopes are used in soluble inorganic form; later, I shall discuss attempts to develop organic compounds incorporating radioactive isotopes – usually either tritium (radioactive hydrogen, ^{3}H) or ^{131}I – as radioactive drugs, as a possible new approach to the chemotherapy of cancer, which I have called radio-chemotherapy (Mitchell, 1968).

In the last 25 years, there has been a remarkable development of the chemotherapy of cancer and allied diseases, largely because of the limitations of surgery and radiotherapy and encouraged by the success of antibacterial chemotherapy. It is stated (Lee Clark, 1961) that 'The use of chemotherapy against cancer was given its greatest impetus during World War II on the physiologic effects of the war gases – sulfur and nitrogen mustards'. Quite apart from this, mention must be made of the study of urethane by Haddow and Sexton (1946) and the classical work of Farber *et al.*

(1948) showing that temporary remissions could be produced in acute leukaemia in children by the folic acid antagonist, 4-amino-pteroyl-glutamic acid (aminopterin). Subsequently, there has been intense interest in this field throughout the world. 'In the United States alone, through the Cancer Chemotherapy National Service Center, an annual budget of about $30,000,000 a year is specifically allocated to produce drugs and test them for anti-cancer activity in animals and man' (Karnofsky, 1964). May I add that the National Cancer Institute in Bethesda prepares and distributes free the very useful 'Cancer Chemotherapy Reports'. One has the impression that during the last few years, the use of chemotherapy in the palliative treatment of patients with advanced, recurrent and generalised malignant disease has improved to some extent, e.g. for carcinoma of the ovary, although there are many disappointments in this field. Treatment is often limited by the toxicity of the drugs; fortunately this is not often the case for steroids, e.g. in some advanced cases of reticulum cell sarcoma treated with Prednisone by mouth, complete remissions have been obtained for several years. It is interesting that a controlled trial of the treatment of patients with chronic myeloid leukaemia showed chemotherapy with busulphan (Myleran) was superior to radiotherapy. (*Report of the M R C's Working Party for Therapeutic Trials in Leukaemia*, 1968); however, this treatment is only palliative, though useful, and not curative in the sense of complete destruction of leukaemic cells. Many new chemotherapeutic agents, and various combinations of agents have been investigated. It is clear that much more effective chemotherapeutic agents are needed. Perhaps the increasing knowledge of molecular biology will contribute to their development. It seems to me that macromolecular chemotherapeutic agents should be investigated. One of the most important developments is the finding that chemotherapy can apparently cure a substantial proportion of women with the rare and biologically unique but very serious gestational tumour, chorio-carcinoma, even after extensive metastases have formed. (Hertz *et al.*, 1958; Hertz,

1967; Bagshawe, 1969). For this purpose, the most important chemotherapeutic agents are amethopterin (Methotrexate), Actinomycin D, Vinblastine, and 6-mercaptopurine. Bagshawe (1968) of Fulham Hospital, London, reported on 150 patients with chorio-carcinoma and other trophoblastic proliferations treated by chemotherapy, sometimes in combinations with surgery, radiotherapy and immunotherapy during the previous ten years. 'The overall permanent remission rate for gestational tumours is 82% and for morphologically confirmed gestational carcinoma it is 70%'.

Mention must also be made of a number of clinical investigations in progress to try to prevent the formation and development of metastases by means of chemotherapy, both during the operation and post-operatively even for long periods. There is some evidence that a small but useful improvement of survival can be obtained in early cases of carcinoma of the bronchus post-operatively with a series of courses of chemotherapy with Cyclophosphamide (Karrer, 1964). However, there is conflicting evidence in this field and much further work is necessary.

One of the problems of the chemotherapy of cancer is that the choice of the agents is largely empirical. In recent years and at the present time, attempts are being made to select the best chemotherapeutic agents and hormones and related compounds for use in the individual case by *in vitro* tests on primary short-term cultures of the tumour cells (Cobb, Walker and Wright, 1961) or on organ cultures of specimens of tumours. My colleague, Dr P. Dendy, has been carrying out and investigating the problem by means of tests on short-term cultures of tumour cells freshly grown from operation and biopsy specimens and ascitic fluid, following the methods developed by Limburg and Krahe (1964). So far, Dr Dendy has cultured over 400 specimens, particularly from cases of carcinoma of the ovary (Dendy, 1968; Dendy, Bozman and Wheeler, 1970). Up to 15 drugs including hormones have been tested but the most striking responses in ovarian carcinoma have been obtained with only one, or sometimes two of the following agents: Melphalan, Trenimon, Cyclophosphamide (Endoxan), Thiotepa, Prednisolone, Progesterone, Vinblastin and Chlorambucil. The test has shown that although some tumours respond with growth inhibition to Prednisolone (phosphate), the growth in certain cases appears to be stimulated by Prednisolone. Moreover, after a time, the clinical response of tumours to the selected chemotherapeutic agents may change. So far, on the basis of survival times, the results with advanced cases of carcinoma of the ovary are very interesting (cf. Limburg, 1968). Another approach is to study the inhibition by drugs of the incorporation of tritium-labelled uridine and thymidine into slices of tumour, incubated aerobically, by means of autoradiography (Oates, 1968). All these developments must be examined very critically. Many of these methods do not take into account the host-tumour relationships and probably the clinical validity of the results can be assessed only after many years. Similar studies of radiation response have not been successful.

However, the investigation of the biological characteristics of tumours in different individual patients, and of differences between primary and secondary tumours, is an approach which must be developed, particularly in relation to biochemical behaviour in a wide sense, including molecular biology. It is my view that this general approach is one of the best ways, not only to improve the treamtent of individual patients but to overcome the serious difficulty of the lack of fundamental knowledge about cancer, particularly in man.

II

Assessment of the results of treatment

Although different types of cancer respond very differently to treatment, it is interesting to start with the survival figures for all the cases of malignant disease in a particular geographical area. In all these considerations, 'rodent ulcer' – basal cell carcinoma of the skin – will be excluded to avoid bias because it usually responds very well to treatment and the survival figures give no real indication of the success of the treatment; e.g. in the East Anglian region 190 out of 214 cases of basal cell carcinoma in all stages of the disease survived 5 years, i.e. with a crude survival rate of 89·2% – not corrected for age or deaths from intercurrent disease. The only recent and reasonably complete data easily available are the crude 5-year survival figures collected by Cancer Registries. The 1968 Annual Report of the South Western Cancer Records Bureau, Bristol and Plymouth, gives information about the follow-up of all the cases of malignant growths, excluding rodent ulcer, registered by doctors and records staffs of hospitals in the year 1961. There were 7,430 cases registered, 5,265 treated and 1,806 alive after 5 years; thus, of the cases registered 24·3% survived 5 years and of the cases treated 34·3%. Similar figures for the East Anglian region for the year 1963, when 4,801 cases were registered and 1,133 of these received no treatment, were 21·9% 5-year survivals for the cases registered and 29·8% for those treated (Cancer Records Bureau, Cambridge, 1969).

It is very difficult to obtain earlier figures which are even approximately comparable. Reference must be made first to the results of a very complete and critical investigation in Sweden for the years 1911–13, carried out by the Swedish Cancer Society (Nyström, 1922). The data presented show that of 7,754 cases of all types of malignant disease registered, excluding cancer of the skin but including melanoma, approximately 9·4% survived 5 years after treatment – which was mainly surgical, although radiotherapy was advanced at that time. A later investigation of great interest is the Survey of Cancer in London, carried out by the British Empire Cancer Campaign (Harnett, 1952) and dealing with cases of malignant disease registered for both out-patients and in-patients in the years 1938 and 1939 by the staffs of the Voluntary and L C C Hospitals and of most of the special hospitals in the County of London. Excluding the 716 cases of rodent ulcer, there were 13,466 primary cases, of which 2,263 were alive 5 years, i.e. 16·8% of the registered cases; 3,260 patients were not treated, so that the 5-year survival rate for those treated was 22·2%. In this whole group, only 322 patients were untraced despite the disorganisation due to the war. Unfortunately, it is not possible to estimate the number of cases not referred to hospitals and the population from which the cases were drawn was not clearly defined. It seems likely that the survival rate for the registered cases is an overestimate for the corresponding population as a whole.

The comparison of these older crude overall survival rates with the recent data from cancer registries is obviously subject to considerable error. However, the figures related to the numbers of cases registered appear to give strong support to the view that there has been a slow improvement in the overall results of the treatment of large numbers of patients with all types of cancer, excluding rodent ulcer. I think it is interesting that in the East Anglian region about 30% of all the patients treated in the year 1963 for malignant diseases, excluding rodent ulcer, which is unusually frequent here, survived 5 years. This is a realistic figure and not over-optimistic. Later, I shall make the point that 5-year survival is not a good measure of cure in many types of cancer. Moreover, it is necessary to draw the serious and sad conclusion that 70% of the patients treated have died within 5 years. At this point, I would like to emphasise that the aim of treatment of patients with cancer – or at least, my aim – is not prolongation of life per se but survival in good health. To estimate the 'quality of life' it is necessary to use some form of Performance Status, such as that of Karnofsky *et al.* (1951); from a practical point of view it has proved to be almost too difficult to follow the course of the Performance Status, except in special investigations. However, may I say that I have the impression that over the last 40 years, there has been an obvious trend in the direction of improved quality of life in patients treated for malignant disease.

However, the value of even the most reliable crude overall 5-year survival figure for all the patients with cancer in a geographically defined region is limited. It is essential to study the results for the treatment of each type of cancer, while noting the great variability usually observed in all aspects of the behaviour of cancer of any particular type in different individual patients. There are two main aspects of this problem: (1) the assessment of the end results of accepted methods of treatment and (2) the evaluation of alternative methods of treatment and particularly of new methods.

For the accepted methods of treatment in routine use, there is a great deal of information about the survival of patients after 5 and 10 years, often including age-corrected survival; it is essential to separate the results for cases where the diagnosis was confirmed histologically. Reference may be made here to '*The Registrar General's Statistical Review of England and Wales for the year 1961: Supplement on Cancer* (1967) which includes results for 1948–49 registrations, and the International Symposium on End Results of Cancer Therapy (Cutler, 1964). As an example one can start with cancer of the gastro-intestinal tract, which is common in both men and women and for which the treatment is still mainly surgical. For all cases registered in England and Wales in 1948–49, the crude 5-year survival rates for men were 9·2% of cancer of the stomach, 27·5% for cancer of the large intestine and 30·6% for cancer of the rectum. Women on the whole do rather better than men. Of the 5-years survivors about two-thirds were alive after a further 5 years; the age-corrected survival rates are of course rather higher. For the patients with localised cancer, the corresponding 5-year crude survival rates for men were for stomach 21·9%, large intestine 45·0% and rectum 43·7%. These and many similar results from other countries emphasise the need for new approaches to treatment and, if possible, to diagnosis at an early stage, especially for cancer of the stomach.

It is usually unwise to try to assess the results of the treatment of patients with cancer with less than 5 years subsequent observation; often longer follow-up for at least 10 and preferably 20 years or even longer is desirable. However, the size of the cured group is usually not immediately obvious from the crude or age-corrected survival figures.

THE CURED GROUP

At this point, I want to state quite clearly that substantial numbers of patients with proven cancer have been cured. Every large department treating cancer has considerable numbers of patients who are alive and well without any recurrence 15 to 20 years and more after treatment of some major form of malignant disease. From the quantitative point of view, it is useful to introduce the concept of the *cured group*, defined as the fraction of those treated which survives as if there had been no cancer, or treatment, and dies at the normal mortality rate for the sex and age and for all cases of death. This definition of cure seems to have been put forward first by Dr Major Greenwood in 1926. Methods of calculating the size of the fraction of the patients who were cured in the sense that they experienced the same life expectancy as that of the normal population have been developed by Boag (1948, 1949), Berkson and Gage (1952) and Haybittle (1959, 1960).

There appears to be strong evidence for the existence of a cured group significantly greater than zero in a number of different types of cancer. For example (see Fig. 1) from the survival curve for the 20-year follow-up of 1,708 cases of cancer of the uterine cervix treated in the years 1925–34 at Radiumhemmet, Stockholm (Kottmeier and Forssner, 1955; Kottmeier, 1962), it

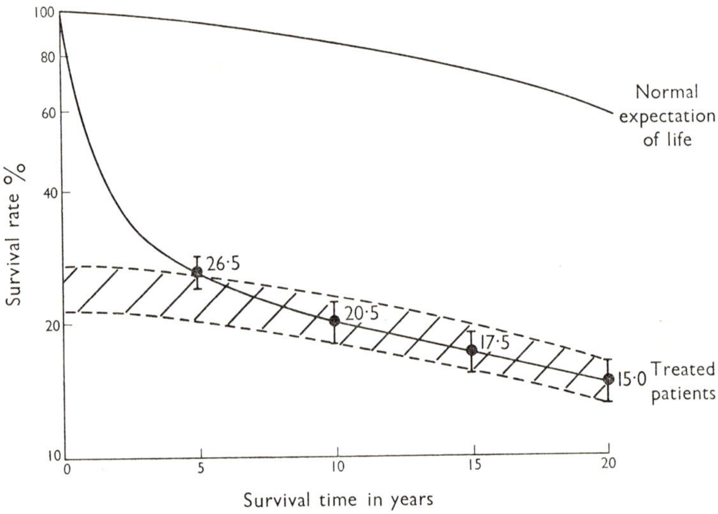

Fig. 1 Survival curve for the 20 year follow-up of 1,708 cases of cancer of the uterine cervix treated in the years 1925–34 at Radiumhemmet, Stockholm (Kottmeier and Forssner, 1955). It was estimated that 24 (±2)% of the patients had a normal life expectancy, as shown in the strip between the dotted lines (Haybittle, 1964).

was estimated that 24 (± 2)% of these patients had a normal life expectancy (Haybittle, 1964). A detailed analysis of a larger group of 4,396 patients treated for carcinoma of the cervix in the years 1914–41, also at Radiumhemmet, showed that among the 1,330 patients apparently well after 5 years, recurrences and metastases and occasionally new cancers at the same site were found in 108 at 5–10 years after treatment, 38 at 10–15 years and 10 at over 15 years (Belonoschkin, 1955); thus 26·7% of the 4,396 patients treated did not die of cancer of the cervix. Nevertheless, the problem is difficult and different types of cancer may behave differently. For example, Cutler and Axtell (1963) found that the 'long survivors' among 254 women with localised cancer of the breast had a mortality about 2½ times normal, but on the other hand, the data of Brinkley and Haybittle (1968) appear to be consistent with a genuinely cured group with no increase in mortality. In this study of the results of a 15-year follow-up of 704 female patients with cancer of the breast, who were treated in Cambridge in the years 1947–50, inclusive, the cured group was estimated at 20·2 ± 2·7%. For the 305 cases in the earlier stages – I and II – the proportion cured is estimated at 26·0 ± 4·7%, while for the 291 cases in the late stages – III and IV – the proportion cured is only 5·3 ± 2·1%. The numbers of cases are relatively small. It is interesting that the results of treatment of 6,775 cases in stages I and II published by Bond (1968) are consistent with an estimate of the proportion cured of 26·4 ± 1·7% (Haybittle, 1968). The data for follow-up for 15 to 25 years suggest that the method of calculation used may *under*-estimate the size of the cured group. These conclusions reflect the seriousness of the problems but nevertheless do *not* support the fatalistic view that cancer of the breast can never be cured by present methods. Despite the difficulties, it would seem wise at the present time to do every thing possible to improve the detection of cancer of the breast at an early stage. However, it must be emphasised that the growth of distant metastases is the commonest cause of failure to cure patients with cancer of the breast. It is clear that much further investigation of the problems of this disease is an urgent necessity.

An interesting and entirely different approach has been made to the problem of estimating cure by Collins, Loeffler and Tivey (1956). In the case of tumours in children, the time taken for the primary tumour to grow to a detectable size cannot be greater than the nine months *in utero* plus the age of the child when the tumour was first observed. If it is assumed that any recurrence after treatment grows at the same rate as did the primary tumour, the recurrence should be observed within a period after treatment equal to the age when the tumour was observed plus 9 months; thus, if no recurrence has appeared within twice the age at which the tumour was detected plus 9 months, the child can be regarded as cured. Although the method of approach presents problems (see Marsden and Steward, 1968, p. 245) and a few exceptions have been reported, the value of Collins' rule appears to be supported by the evidence for Wilms' tumour (Collins, 1958), neuroblastoma (Knox and Kingsley Pillers, 1958) and medulloblastoma (Bloom, Wallace and Henk, 1969).

INVESTIGATION OF NEW METHODS OF TREATMENT

The assessment of the clinical value of any new form of treatment of cancer proves almost invariably to be much more difficult than might be expected. The main reasons for this are the great variability in the natural history and behaviour of apparently similar malignant tumours in different patients, the differences in the physical and mental response of the individual patients to their disease and to the treatment and often the length of time necessary to evaluate the results of treatment. In order to assess the value of a particular method of treatment, it is usually essential to consider the results for large numbers of patients. Only rarely are the results of a new method of treatment of cancer so striking and so consistent that its advantages appear to be immediately obvious and generally acceptable. This was the case with megavoltage radiations. In addition to the theoretical advantages arising from their physical properties, it quickly became clear that treatment by means of ^{60}Co γ-radiations and high energy X-rays is usually easier to carry out and considerably more comfortable for the patients than conventional deep X-ray therapy. The general introduction of megavoltage radiotherapy without planned clinical trials or survival studies with long-term follow-up emphasises the fact that the acceptance of a new method of treatment is essentially a matter of conviction, based on ordinary clinical observation and common sense. However, in most cases, where the new treatment produces only a relatively small improvement of the results, this approach can lead, only too easily, to serious errors in the decisions concerning both the acceptance and the rejection of new methods of treatment.

In general, the evaluation of new methods of treatment of cancer presents substantial and often very difficult problems. Historically, an important example is the treatment of cancer of the uterine cervix. It is salutary to recall that in the original investigations of the use of radium (and mesothorium), it took 10 years – from 1903 to 1913 – before the value of the method in technically operable cases was recognised (see Ries and Breitner, 1959). The earliest attempts to use X-ray therapy were unsuccessful (Deutsch, 1904). It became clear that good results could be obtained only by using sufficiently large amounts of radium (Abbé, 1904; Döderlein, 1913). Only after another 10–15 years were the five-year results published for a number of large independent series of cases of carcinoma of the cervix treated by radiotherapy (see Forssell, 1928, p. 30). As is widely known, the subsequent study of the treatment of carcinoma of the cervix is a field in which there has been valuable and effective international co-operation. Starting in 1937, with an interruption due to the War, a series of 14 volumes of Annual Reports were published from the Editorial Office in Stockholm (Kottmeier, 1967), analysing statements of the results of treatment from 124 institutions in 26 countries and including a total of 262,548 examined cases of carcinoma of the cervix. However, even with this evidence from over a quarter of a million patients, there are still admissible differences of opinion about the right lines of treatment. It is important to note that it is not possible to formulate a generally acceptable policy concerning the indications for surgery and radiotherapy in individual patients. As emphasised by the late Professor J. Heyman of Stockholm, it must be concluded that to a large extent, experience of the method of treatment used is more important than the method itself, provided that this is a good one.

CLINICAL TRIALS

It is obviously essential to develop methods for reaching a reliable conclusion about the value of any method of treatment of cancer in as short a time as possible. In recent years, a tremendous effort has been devoted to clinical trials, particularly of new drugs but also of different methods of surgery, radiotherapy and chemotherapy and of various combinations of these. The need for properly designed trials of any new methods of treatment was emphasised by their use in the clinical evaluation of chemotherapeutic agents in tuberculosis (Medical Research Council, 1948, 1950). In general, from a statistical point of view, the basic principles of clinical trials are now well understood, largely as a result of the classical studies by R. A. Fisher (1925, 1935) of the design of agricultural and biological experiments and of the pioneer work of A. Bradford Hill (1952) on the design of clinical trials. Nevertheless, agricultural, biological and industrial experiments differ in a number of ways from clinical trials. Many difficult and serious problems are encountered in the practical design, conduct and analysis of acceptable clinical trials of new methods of treatment of patients with cancer (see e.g. Mitchell, 1960; Marrian, Marshall and Mitchell, 1961; Brinkley and Haybittle, 1965; Deeley, 1967). Moreover, there appear to be unresolved theoretical difficulties, when as often happens, relatively small numbers of cases are involved (Wrighton, 1953). It is easy with reasonable assumptions, to calculate the number of patients required in each of two treatment groups, which are being compared, in order to have a 90% chance of detecting a difference at the 5% level of significance (Patnaik, 1948; Bankier and Batley, 1957). For example, to improve the survival rate from 25% with the 'old' treatment to 40% with the 'new method' 199, say 200 patients are required in each treatment group, while for the much more important example of 5% improvement, 1,605 patients are needed in each group. However, the problem of the numbers of cases required in a particular clinical trial is often difficult; it may be desirable to accept a lower chance of detecting a difference at the 5% level of significance (see also Boag, 1960). It is interesting that in reviewing the results of 25 clinical trials involving radiotherapy, Graffman and Jung (1970) have calculated the differences that would have been regarded as significant at the 5% level with a probability of 50% and of 95% for the numbers of patients in the particular trial. They conclude that 'of the order of 1,000 patients should be entered in each group of a clinical trial if the difference that can be expected is to be demonstrated significantly with a fair probability'. In general, these numbers can be obtained in a reasonable length of time such as one year or two years at the most, only by the co-operation of a number of centres. Nevertheless, it is in any case usually wise to start with a 'pilot trial' (Mitchell 1960, p. 160). Statistical methods can be regarded as a kind of insurance. One general problem is the level of statistical significance which is chosen for protection against the error of recommending the 'new' treatment when, in fact, it is no better than the 'old' method. The level of significance widely used is the traditional 5%. However, it has been suggested (e.g. Bross, 1952) that in many trials, a 10% (i.e. 1 in 10) risk of erroneously recommending a new treatment is acceptable. My view is that there are circumstances where this is justified but that this is a difficult problem, particularly when it is argued that the treatment of large numbers of patients will be influenced by the decision. Moreover, clinical impressions can be misleading.

It is useful to quote from a recent lecture by Sir Austin Bradford Hill (1970) on the power and limitations of statistical methods in connection with controlled clinical trials: 'There is one limitation I would stress – not of the method but of the reasoning of the user and consumer. This is an exaggerated respect for tests of significance . . . .' and 'A very true criticism of the controlled trial is that it usually tells us that *on the average* treatment A gives better results than treatment B. It rarely tells us that treatment A is the method of choice for Mr Smith'.

There are usually patients who do not respond to a particular form of treatment. In setting up a clinical trial it is desirable to record a great many possibly relevant findings for each individual patient before treatment. In doing this, clinical experience and judgment are absolutely essential. The analysis of the large amount of evidence which should be collected is made possible by the use of computers, so that there should now be much greater opportunities to determine the factors involved in response or lack of response to treatment.

In the investigation of any new method of treatment of cancer, one must start with a preliminary trial to see whether it is worth further study and if this appears to be the case, then continue the exploratory phase of the trial to estimate the effectiveness of the method and in the case of a drug, to obtain information about optimal dosage. In quantitative terms, Gehan (1961) showed that if the drug were effective in 20% of patients, or more, there would be a 95% chance of one or more 'successes' in 14 consecutive cases. Taking as an example, our own attempt in Cambridge to develop a radioactive drug ('tritiated MNDP') for use in patients with advanced and recurrent cancer (Mitchell, 1965a), there were five 'responses' – which were estimated on the modest basis of reduction in size of the tumour or part of the tumour – in the first 14 cases. It was then necessary to study a further 86 cases in order to estimate a therapeutic effectiveness of 20% with a standard error of $\pm$ 5%. In fact, it was found that among the first 102 cases (including the initial 14), there were 16 responses. Among these cases, the difference between the results after administration of the higher and of the lower total doses was statistically highly significant; ($P<0{\cdot}001$). Accordingly, the second phase of the trial was continued, to work out the indications for the new method and the practical details of dosage (see below). The third phase involves the treatment of selected patients with clearly defined indications; at this stage of the investigation, some estimate of the value of the drug should be emerging.

In many new developments, it is necessary at some stage to compare the effectiveness of the new agent or method with that of a generally accepted and widely used procedure. For this purpose and with suitable and carefully considered safeguards, the most efficient method is the use of the designed trial with random allocation of patients and statistical assessment, as already mentioned. Proper initial design of the trial is absolutely essential. The basis of our own trials of this type in Cambridge has been the comparison of two, or more, forms of treatment. One of these is already widely used and the other, or others, can be regarded as new but supported by sufficient preliminary evidence to suggest that there is a real prospect of improvement of the new form of treatment. It must be emphasised that every patient receives individual treatment which is either standard practice or can be expected to give results which are at least as good and possibly better. My view is that a patient should *only* be put into a randomised trial, when one honestly does not know which is the best method of treatment for the particular individual patient. I think that none of those of us who are involved in clinical trials minimises the responsibility to the individual patients under our care. I feel very strongly that the use of untreated control patients cannot be contemplated. I also consider that it is necessary in the interests of patients to plan to be able to depart, when required, from what may be termed the theoretically ideal form of 'experiment' with deliberate sacrifice of information; e.g. if a patient is allocated to one form of treatment and the doctor responsible decides that it is better or preferable to give the other form of treatment, this is of course given but the patient is assessed for the form of treatment that was originally allocated. It is vital that, in considering numbers, one never loses sight of the individual patient and his or her welfare. The degree of responsibility involved in the design of clinical trials and in their conduct, often over many years is sometimes almost unendurable. The ethical problems of therapeutic trials of new forms of treatment of patients with cancer are serious enough but they appear to me to be usually less difficult than those of non-therapeutic clinical research, which have been considered in the Declaration of Helsinki (1962) and in the *Report of the Medical Research Council* for 1962–63 (1964); see also Dr Pappworth's book *Human Guinea-pigs* (1967).

It is worth mentioning, though perhaps obvious, that a patient should only be put into a trial, when all the strictly defined clinical and pathological criteria specified in the design of the trial are satisfied, otherwise dilution by unsuitable cases reduces the significance of the results.

The criteria for the assessment of the results of treatment must be as objective as possible. It is clear that cure rate or 5-year survival rate or disease-free rate is desirable as a criterion for the assessment of the long-term results. However, this is usually not practicable where the aim of the treatment is essentially palliative. In these circumstances survival times from the beginning (or end) of treatment and also from the first symptom are of great value; after considering various alternative criteria, one usually comes back to rely on these. It must be mentioned that for patients who are not cured, the logarithms of the survival times are usually distributed approximately normally (Boag, 1948, 1960; Kaufmann, 1966; Lenarduzzi, Valdagni and Pistolesi, 1967). Accordingly, it is desirable to estimate the mean log survival time (Mitchell, Brinkley and Haybittle, 1965). However, it is also desirable to try to include assessment of what is now called the 'quality of life', using some form of Performance Status (see Karnofsky *et al.*, 1951; Mitchell, 1960) and also to take account of the complications of treatment. It is important to know what the patient feels about the treatment and whether the patient was pleased with the treatment. One suspects that further theoretical studies might be rewarding, e.g. concerning the problem of types of cases included in the trial, which do not respond to treatment, although this was not recognised beforehand (see Healey and Anderson, 1965).

It seems to me that insufficient attention has been paid to the problem of deciding when to stop a randomised clinical trial of the treatment of patients with cancer. We have tried sequential methods of various types (see Wald, 1947; Bross, 1952; Armitage, 1954, 1960; Mitchell, 1960; Brinkley and Haybittle, 1965), but all our trials have, in fact, stopped when the doctors taking part felt that the new method was better than the standard procedure (see e.g. Mitchell, 1960; p. 160; Marrian, Marshall and Mitchell, 1961, p. 262; Brinkley and Haybittle, 1966). One cannot do otherwise and must use the new method for all the patients for which it is suitable, even though in some instances the evidence is not conclusive.

From a practical point of view, designed clinical trials involve a large amount of work and persistent effort often over many years, with careful organisation which is particularly necessary since enthusiasm for this difficult and often trying type of activity decreases rapidly. In future, co-operation between a number of centres is likely to be essential in order to treat sufficiently large numbers of patients, perhaps 600–1,000 in each of two treatment groups, in a short time such as one year or at the most two years. The late Sir Henry Dale once said that 'medical research is largely drudgery'; I know from experience that this is true for clinical trials. Nevertheless, although it is essential to be critical, evidence which is impressive has been obtained in a number of clinical trials, where previous retrospective studies had given answers which were either inconclusive or not convincing.

The treatment of the earlier 'operable' stages of cancer of the breast provides an important example. Since Halsted introduced his classical operation of radical mastectomy in 1894, it has generally been regarded as the standard treatment of 'early' cancer of the breast. Until relatively recently, various attempts to introduce lesser techniques have met with disapproval. Even in 1928, Burton J. Lee of New York reported on the treatment of primary operable cancer of the breast 'by irradiation alone or in conjunction with conservative surgery'. In 1941, a major contribution was made by Professor R. McWhirter (1955) of Edinburgh, by the use of simple mastectomy and post-operative X-ray therapy instead of radical mastectomy. Despite the apparently convincing results, this method was widely criticised. However, in 1951, Kaae and Johansen (1968) started a randomised trial at the Radium Centre in Copenhagen; this continued until 1957 and included 666 patients. In 1967, they reported the 10-year results of their trial, which show that the results of treatment by means of simple mastectomy followed by post-operative X-ray therapy are essentially the same as those of treatment by an extended radical mastectomy without supplementary irradiation. Quite independently, following our survey of the results of treatment of all cases of cancer of the breast in Cambridge (see Brinkley and Haybittle, 1959), we started a trial of the treatment of Stage II cases of cancer of the female breast, with the co-operation of eight surgeons in the area and with particular encouragement from Mr B. McN. Truscott. Radical mastectomy was compared with modified simple mastectomy, each in combination with the same technique of post-operative X-ray therapy. The trial was started in October 1958 and finished in May 1965, and included 204 patients. The present conclusion from the results of this trial published by Dr D. M. Brinkley and Dr J. L. Haybittle (1966) is that, in the treatment of Stage II carcinoma of the breast by surgery and standard post-operative X-ray therapy, a *modified simple mastectomy* is preferable to a radical operation. 'A modified simple mastectomy consisted in the removal of the breast tissue without the removal of the pectoral muscle. It might include removal of accessible axillary glands, but there was no block dissection of the axilla'. In fact among the 113 patients in the simple group, 89 had lymph nodes removed. Dr Brinkley and Dr Haybittle have kindly made the most recent information concerning survival rates and recurrence-free rates available to me for this lecture. The results for all the patients in the trial, for those patients with tumours of histological grade II, i.e. of medium malignancy and for those with histological evidence of carcinoma in axillary nodes are given in Table I. It must be emphasised that none of the differences at 5 or 10 years is statistically significant. However, continued long-term follow-up of the patients is essential. There appeared to be significantly higher

Table I. *Cambridge trial of the treatment of Stage II carcinoma of the breast*

Comparison of radical mastectomy with modified simple mastectomy, each in combination with the same technique of post-operative X-ray therapy. Results assessed at 30.6.69

		No. of cases	5 years Survival rate	5 years Recurrence-free rate	10 years Survival rate	10 years Recurrence-free rate
All patients	Radical	91	61·2±5·2	53·7±5·3	54·8±5·6	46·2±5·9
	Simple	113	64·1±4·6	58·2±4·7	44·8±5·7	41·3±5·4
Grade II tumours	Radical	63	63·7±6·2	55·7±6·4	54·3±6·9	44·8±7·3
	Simple	60	58·9±6·5	56·2±6·5	47·5±7·5	40·4±7·7
Positive axillary glands	Radical	53	47·1±7·0	37·9±6·8	38·4±7·4	25·3±7·1
	Simple	50	47·6±7·1	37·9±6·9	32·2±7·2	28·0±6·6

survival and recurrence-free rates after 5 years in the modified simple mastectomy group for the relatively small numbers of patients with histologically positive axillary nodes and no skin tethering and/or dimpling. Of greater interest is the reduced morbidity in the modified simple mastectomy group, with significantly less delay in healing ($P<0{\cdot}01$) than after the radical operation. It was this finding in association with the preliminary survey of our results in 1965, together with the results obtained by Kaae and Johansen (1965), which made us feel that the likelihood of the radical operation offering any advantage was very small; accordingly, entry into the trial was then stopped.

At the present time, it seems that a useful step forward has been achieved by means of the clinical trials which have shown the value of simple or modified simple mastectomy in suitable cases instead of some form of radical mastectomy. However, a number of other trials involving radical mastectomy are still being carried out or planned. On the other hand, there is considerable doubt about the value of post-operative radiotherapy in operable cases of cancer of the breast and also a possibility of harmful effects in some circumstances (cf. Bond, 1970). It is to be noted that Easson (1968) of Manchester found essentially the same survival rates over 10 years after treatment for 750 patients in whom the initial treatment was radical mastectomy only – X-ray therapy being reserved for recurrence – and for 707 patients in whom radical mastectomy was combined with post-operative X-ray therapy. This is a difficult problem and dose and time factors may be important. A new trial, initiated by groups at Addenbrooke's Hospital, Cambridge, and King's College Hospital, London, and involving the collaboration of a number of centres in the U.K. has been started on 1 April 1970; the aim is to compare the value of simple, or extended simple mastectomy together with post-operative regional radiotherapy with that of similar conservative surgery alone, without any other treatment unless active recurrent disease appears, in female patients with carcinoma of the breast, in general, in both Stages I and II, or more precisely T1N0 and T2N0 and T1N1 and T2N1 (M0), respectively (*Lancet*, 1969). However, it is likely that any dramatic improvement in the results can come only from fundamentally new approaches.

III

Development of research in relation to radiotherapy

Turning now to laboratory research in relation to the radiotherapy of malignant tumours in patients, it is perhaps simplest to introduce the rather detailed consideration of certain aspects of the work of my colleagues and myself in Cambridge by summarising briefly the development of the main lines of thought and investigation.

In my own early work, a disturbance of nucleic acid metabolism with accumulation of 'pentose nucleotides' and RNA and inhibition of synthesis of DNA – which was considered in relation to mitotic inhibition – was demonstrated, mainly in human tumours after therapeutic doses of radiation, by the use of ultraviolet photomicrography combined with photographic photometry and histochemical studies (Mitchell, 1940, 1942a b, c, 1943, 1944). This work led me to suggest that the killing of tumour cells in radiotherapy was based on the production of what I called a 'macromolecular lesion' of DNA in the nucleoprotein system of the nucleus of the living cell (Mitchell, 1955, 1956; see also 1960). This attempt to identify the radiosensitive target biochemically was essentially a transition from the classical target theory of radiobiological action to molecular radiobiology, though I did not think of it in these terms at that time.

The demonstration of the production of a far-reaching biochemical disturbance by ionizing radiations suggested the possibility of radiosensitisation by chemical agents. I and my colleagues have worked on this problem since 1946, particularly with Synkavit (Roche Products Ltd), 2-methyl-1,4-naphthaquinol-bis-(disodium phosphate), abbreviated here MNDP (see Fig. 2), which I selected on the basis of its molecular structure and low toxicity (see Mitchell, 1948) – though in some details the reasoning was probably not correct.

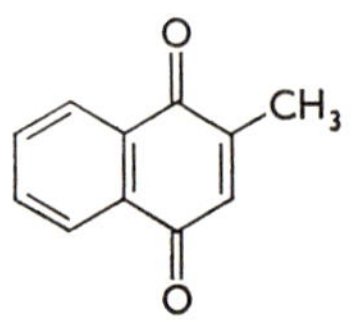

2-methyl-1,4-naphthaquinone
(menadione)

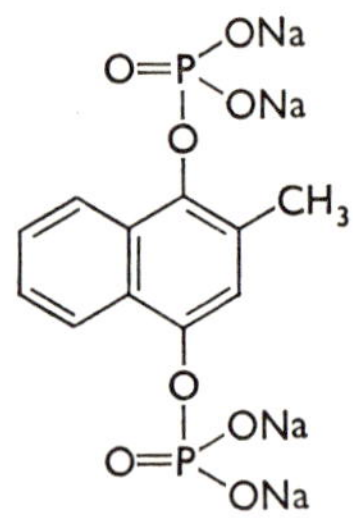

2-methyl-1,4-naphthaquinol
bis(disodium phosphate), MNDP, (Synkavit)

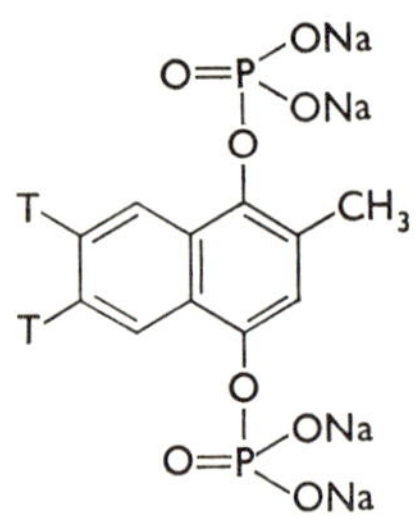

The radioactive drug TRK 219
2-methyl-6,7-ditritio-1,4-
naphthaquinol bis(disodium phosphate)

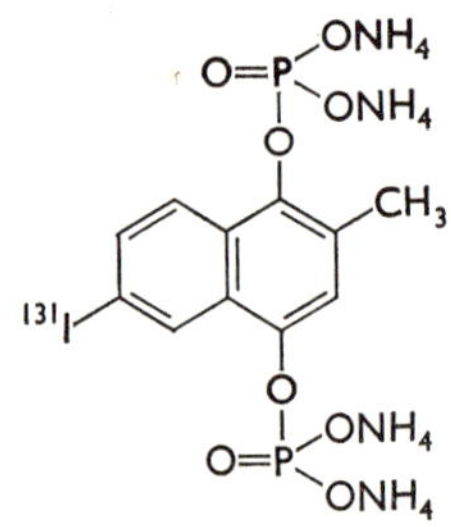

6-^{131}I-iodo-MNDP

Fig. 2 Formulae of the most important compounds.

This compound had the advantage that it was already in use in medicine as a synthetic vitamin K substitute, though comparison of the biological effects of a series of related compounds showed that the mitotic inhibiting action had no association with vitamin K activity (Mitchell and Simon-Reuss, 1952). It may be of interest to mention that although 340 compounds were tested, Synkavit, which was the first compound studied, still appears to be the best. From a practical point of view, and with the exception of one clinical trial, the clinical results have been in general modest or negative. However, the investigations have proved to be of considerable scientific interest, particularly in relation to radiation chemistry and the study of the general problem of radiosensitisation by a wide range of chemical agents.*

Further, going back to 1946, when we first started to investigate Synkavit as a radiosensitiser, we noticed with some patients that at about a minute after intravenous injection of doses of 100-150 mg of Synkavit, there was local pain in the region of the tumour. This purely accidental finding led us to study the selective concentration of Synkavit in tumour cells and to the investigation of the possibliities of radioactive drugs in the treatment and diagnosis of patients with malignant diseases. From the point of view of therapy, we have developed tritiated derivatives of MNDP of very high specific activity and for tumour localisation and possible diagnostic applications, the radio-iodine labelled derivative, 6-^{131}I-iodo-MNDP. We have also studied some other compounds, including tritiated Atebrin (Young, 1963; Young, Wild and Simon-Reuss, 1965) and tritiated ubiquinone derivatives (Birdsall, 1967).

Over the years, in addition to pursuing what is now sometimes called 'mission oriented research', I have always tried to devote a major part of the limited effort available to 'fundamental' investigations.

SOME WORK IN PROGRESS OF BOTH CLINICAL AND SCIENTIFIC INTEREST

(i) *Radiosensitisers*

The idea of improving the selective response of malignant tumours to therapeutic irradiation by means of chemical agents started in the early days of radiology with the work of Werner of Heidelberg in 1905 with a preparation of choline borate (Enzytol). A subject which is closely inter-related with the use of chemical

* Synkavit is best described as the precursor of a radiosensitiser, the quinone, menadione, which acts under anoxic conditions. (O. C. A. Scott, 1971, personal communication.)

radiosensitisers is the role of oxygen. In 1921 Holthusen discovered that the radiosensitivity of Ascaris eggs in an atmosphere of nitrogen was only one-third of that in air. However, despite the work of Fischer-Wasels (1930), Crabtree and Cramer (1933, 1934) and Lacassagne (1942) and the beginnings of the practical use of blood transfusions to improve oxygenation in radiotherapy in 1938, it was not until the publication of the experiments of Thoday and Read (1947) using root-tips of the broad bean, Vicia faba, that the importance of oxygen in increasing radiosensitivity became generally recognised. An important influence subsequently was the work of L. H. Gray and his colleagues, especially O. C. A. Scott (Gray, 1957). Oxygen is the most important radiosensitiser known; as shown by pulse-irradiation studies, it must be present *during* the irradiation (Adams, 1967). It has been widely accepted that radio-resistant anoxic tumour cells are the most important cause of failure to cure many human tumours by radiotherapy. However, there are many problems in this field, including the finding of reoxygenation of anoxic cells after irradiation in some types of both transplantable and spontaneous tumours in mice (van Putten, 1968; van Putten and Kallman, 1968; Begg, Denekamp and Howes, 1969); these results are almost certainly relevant to the choice of the intervals between the individual doses in fractionated radiotherapy, especially in combination with hyperbaric oxygen. It seems to be confirmed that relatively less complete depopulation of the malignant cells by irradiation is necessary to cure localised spontaneous human tumours than most transplantable tumours in mice. Apart from the question of the role of host and immune responses, many early human tumours behave in relation to radiotherapy as if the malignant cells are well oxygenated. Although defective nutrition may increase to some extent the radiosensitivity of populations of tumour cells growing under difficulties (Madoc-Jones, 1964; Hahn, 1968), it now appears reasonably certain that the most important factor limiting the radiocurability of advanced human tumours is the presence of anoxic but viable malignant cells. The studies of hyperbaric oxygen in radiotherapy with X- and γ-rays and of the use of fast neutrons are attempts to circumvent this difficulty. However, if a suitable compound could be found, it would be much simpler to use a radiosensitising drug, which if possible sensitised anoxic malignant cells selectively in relation both to euoxic malignant cells and to normal cells.

Radiosensitisation by chemical agents is now an extensive field of study, mainly in relation to radiation chemistry, radiobiology and radiotherapy, but also in connection with the sterilisation of foods by irradiation; may I refer to reviews by Adams (1967, 1968), Bridges (1969), Foye (1967), Mitchell (1967, 1968b) and Vermund and Gollin (1968), to the review by Scotte Doggett, Bagshaw and Kaplan (1967) dealing with the combined therapy of cancer using chemotherapeutic agents and radiotherapy, and also to the Proceedings of the Second International Symposium on Radiosensitising and Radioprotective Drugs, 1969 (Moroson and Quintiliani, 1970).

Experimental work in this whole area of study appears to be singularly difficult. Different workers often obtain divergent results, presumably because of unrecognised differences in the experimental conditions. It is relevant to note that large differences exist in enzyme activities, e.g. of alkaline phosphatase among different strains of HeLa cells, derived from a case of carcinoma of the cervix (Cox and Griffin, 1967) and of glycerol-3-phosphate dehydrogenase (E.C.1.1.1.8) among different strains of the widely used Ehrlich ascites carcinoma of the mouse (Letnansky, 1968). However, after 25 years work, it can be concluded that the radiosensitivity of some cells can be increased by factors of at least two by certain chemical agents and in some circumstances under anoxic conditions.

It is interesting that many chemical radiosensitisers are sulfhydryl-binding reagents (Bridges, 1969). However, Adams, Cooke and Michael (1968) showed by means of rapid mixing techniques used in conjunction with pulse-irradiation studies that, e.g. with N-ethylmaleimide, radiosensitisation of the bacterium *Serratia marcescens* occurred at times shorter than those required for thermal reactions with -SH groups in the cell. Further study of this problem is necessary.

Among the different chemical types of radiosensitisers, the halogenated pyrimidine analogues (Zamenhof, De Giovanni and Greer, 1958) are of great interest. The demonstration that incorporation of the thymidine analogues, 5-bromo- and 5-iodo-deoxyuridine into the DNA of human cells in tissue culture before irradiation with X-rays produces radiosensitisation, supports the conclusion that for delayed killing of cells, the principal target is DNA (Szybalski, 1960; Djordjevic and Szybalski, 1960). These results have been generally confirmed and extended. However, the mechanism of action is not simple, as confirmed by pulse and steady-state radiolysis studies of bromouracil-substituted and unsubstituted DNA (Zimbrick, Ward and Myers, 1969). The radiosensitisation by these compounds is independent of the presence of oxygen at the time of irradiation (Kaplan, Zavarine and Earle, 1962; Humphrey, Dewey and Cork, 1963). Many clinical investigations have been carried out (Scotte Doggett, Bagshaw and Kaplan, 1967). Of particular interest is the use of 5-bromo-deoxyuridine, when administered by intra-arterial injection, as a radiosensitiser in the radiotherapy of patients with locally advanced cancer of the head and neck (in conjunction with 5-fluorouracil) (Tanaka and Takahashi, 1970) and with various types of cerebral tumours (Hoshino *et al.*, 1970).

An important recent development is the demonstration of radiosensitisation under anoxic conditions by certain electron acceptors in aqueous solution; this process has been termed electron-affinic sensitisation (Adams, 1967, 1968; Adams and Cooke, 1969). Pulse radiolysis studies suggest that direct ionization of the target molecule produces in the first instance, a positive ion and an electron which, after thermalisation, migrates to some electron-affinic site which may be on the target; then, if a molecule of higher electron affinity were present in the immediate environment, electron transfer to the sensitiser would occur, instead of charge recombination with absence of damage to the target. Irreversible electron transfer to the sensitiser would favour the formation of a free radical on the target molecule. This direct-action model had the advantage of accommodating oxygen in the general class of radiosensitisers. Further, oxygen reacts with many radiation-induced free radicals (Willson, 1970). The role of oxidation of SH groups by oxygen is difficult to assess. It is important also to note that oxygen is a small molecule. However, apart from details of the radiochemical mechanism, compounds which have been shown experimentally to act as radiosensitisers under anoxic conditions mainly in the bacterium *Serratia marcescens* include diacetyl, benzophenone, N-ethylmaleimide (Adams and Dewey, 1963), dimethylfumarate, and indanetrione and effective in lowest concentration 2-methyl-1,4-naphthaquinone (menadione) (Adams, 1967, 1968; Adams and Cooke, 1969). Radiosensitisation of mammalian cells has been demonstrated in tissue cultures for indanetrione (Scott and Sturrock, 1968), methylglyoxal (Ashwood-Smith *et al.*, 1967) and phenylglyoxal (Barnes, Ashwood-Smith and Bridges, 1969) and in a mouse ascites tumour under anoxic conditions for indanetrione (Di Vita and Marrian, 1970).

Menadione (see Fig. 2) is of particular interest because it appears to be the 'active form' of Synkavit (Roche Products Ltd) menadiol sodium diphosphate (U.S.P.) – 2-methyl-1,4-naphthaquinol-bis(disodium phosphate), abbreviated here MNDP – which has been studied extensively since 1946 (Mitchell and Simon-Reuss, 1947) as a radiosensitiser in radiotherapy (Mitchell, 1960, 1965, 1967b; Marrian, Marshall and Mitchell, 1961; Mitchell, Brinkley and Haybittle, 1967; Deeley, 1967; Krishnamurthi, Shanta and Krishnan Nair, 1967; Shanta, Krishnamurthi and Sastri, 1969; Evans and Todd, 1969). A number of workers have not confirmed our results in animal experiments or clinical trials. I think that the main reason for this is that some human malignant tumours and some transplanted and spontaneous tumours in mice and rats do not concentrate MNDP selectively (see Marrian,

Mitchell, Bull, King and Szaz, 1968). A number of clinical trials have concerned the palliative radiotherapy of patients with inoperable carcinoma of the bronchus. Deeley (1967) reported a small effect of Synkavit. Evans and Todd (1969) found no significant effect. We carried out an initial trial of Synkavit and a 'pilot trial' of intravenous Synkavit with oxygen inhaled at atmospheric pressure, together with a trial comparing Synkavit and the 2,3-dimethyl analogue (Compound 28) before setting up our major trial. (Mitchell, 1960, pp. 147–166). The results of the survival studies in this last trial (Mitchell, Brinkley and Haybittle, 1967) for 155 male patients with histologically verified inoperable carcinoma of the bronchus showed a small effect of Synkavit, which was regarded as probably significant ($P = 0{\cdot}05$–$0{\cdot}06$). It now seems likely that many cases of carcinoma of the bronchus do not show a high degree of selective concentration of Synkavit in the tumour cells, so that this disease was not a good choice for testing radiosensitisation, quite apart from the fact that most of these patients die with distant metastases.

It may be of interest to record the findings of a retrospective study of all our histologically verified inoperable male cases of carcinoma of the bronchus without evidence of extrathoracic spread treated in the years 1947–63, inclusive, by means of short-term radiotherapy at the medium palliative level of dosage. The patients in this category received calculated central doses of filtered 220–250 kVp X-rays of 1,500–1,750 'old r', 1,750–2,000 'new R' or 2,000–2,500 R of ^{137}Cs or ^{60}Co gamma radiation, delivered in 7–10 treatments in overall time 8–11 days; for further details of the technique see Mitchell (1960) and Mitchell, Brinkley and Haybittle (1967). This mild form of palliative radiotherapy is usually not curative but does not seriously upset the patients and temporarily increases their well-being. Of the 128 patients treated by this method who received Synkavit as a radiosensitiser, 7 survived with normal activity 5 years or more – with follow-up to 17 years so far in one case. Of the comparable 68 cases treated without Synkavit, none survived 5 years. Among the 7 long survivors, the histology of the tumour was squamous carcinoma in 3 cases and adenocarcinoma in one case and was originally considered to be oat-cell carcinoma in 3 cases, but in two of these was probably poorly differentiated squamous carcinoma. If it can be assumed that these two groups of patients are comparable, the finding of a small number of long-survivors in the group receiving Synkavit is probably significant ($P = 0{\cdot}048$). May I add that in considering the results of treatment of carcinoma of the lung, it is important to consider the histologically verified cases separately. 'Generally, unconfirmed cases show a survival rate significantly inferior to the histologically proved' (Gellé and Leguerinais, 1964).

In our clinical investigations of Synkavit as a radiosensitiser in the radiotherapy of inoperable cases of carcinoma of the bronchus in men, the Dose Enhancement Factor can be estimated at about 1·5 for both short-term and long-term results; i.e. it appears that the effective tumour dose was increased by about 50% by the action of the radiosensitiser (Mitchell, 1960, p. 58; see Eichhorn and Lessel, 1968).

It must be mentioned that no evidence of radiosensitisation was found in a clinical trial of 2-methyl-1,4-naphthaquinone sodium bisulphite ('Vitamin K_3') in the radiotherapy of inoperable cases of carcinoma of the bronchus (Becker, 1965): it was considered that one reason for the negative result could be insufficient accumulation of Vitamin K_3 in the tumour. As we shall discuss, it now seems likely that radiosensitisation is observed only when there is a substantial selective concentration of the 'active form' of the compound used in the malignant cells.

By far the most striking clinical results with Synkavit have been published by the group in Madras (Krishnamurthi *et al.*, 1967; Shanta *et al.*, 1969), for a randomised trial of intravenous Synkavit as a radiosensitiser in the radical ^{60}Co gamma-ray therapy of patients with squamous carcinoma of the mucous membrane of the cheek involving from three-quarters to the whole extent of the cheek. The lesions selected were all deeply infiltrating but had not ulcerated externally. The 5-year disease-free survival rate was 27 out of 70 patients treated with Synkavit and irradiation, 38·6%, but only 15 out of 75 – 20% – in the control group treated by means of irradiation only. This difference is statistically significant (P = 0·023).

The possibility must be considered that nutritional and physiological factors, including the pH in the malignant cells, play a part in the radiosensitisation of tumours by Synkavit. The quantitative aspects of the selective uptake of Synkavit into tumour cells and the distribution of the labelled compound in malignant and normal cells, will be discussed in the next section on radioactive drugs. Here, when considering briefly the mechanism of action of Synkavit, it must be mentioned that the uptake into malignant cells has been found to be approximately constant in the pH range 7·2–8·4 but decreases rapidly below pH 7·0 (Dendy, 1967, 1969; Harrison, 1968). The diphosphate, Synkavit, itself is the 'transport form'. Its uptake into tumour cells appears to depend on dephosphorylation and then probably oxidation of the meandiol formed to the 'active form', which is thought to be menadione (Marrian, 1965; Fisher, 1968). In this field there are many unsolved problems. Dendy (1970) has found that the final uptake of tritiated MNDP (TRK 219 – see the next section) is a two-phase process involving degradation and then subsequent uptake into the cells from the pool of degraded products, which is mainly at first extracellular. In studies of the pH dependence of the dephosphorylation of Synkavit by Ehrlich ascites tumour (EAT) cells *in vitro*, Dr Valerie Fisher (1968) showed that two separate enzymes appear to be involved, an acid phosphatase, with pH optimum at 4·4 and a more active *alkaline phosphatase* with maximum activity at about pH 9·5. Lack of glucose in the medium increases the dephosphorylation of Synkavit but not of ATP. The final amount of dephosphorylation of Synkavit is the same for both EAT cells and mouse liver cells *in vitro* but the EAT cells produce an initial burst of dephosphorylation at between 10 and 30 minutes incubation at 37°C, while the liver cells show a steady linear rate of dephosphorylation. It is interesting that 6-iodo-MNDP is dephosphorylated by EAT cells at about the same rate and to much the same extent as Synkavit in the same molar concentration. Further it may be mentioned that in the earlier tests on chick fibroblast cultures (Mitchell, Simon-Reuss and King, 1960), 6-iodo-MNDP was found to be a radiosensitiser with a value of the Potentiation Factor of slightly less than 2, i.e. about the same as for Synkavit. Although Synkavit itself is not useful as a cancer chemotherapeutic agent, it has been found to produce inhibition of the growth of tumour cells under certain carefully defined experimental conditions. It retards the the growth of mouse ascites tumour cells provided that the pH of the medium during incubation before inoculation was maintained at pH 7·4 (Harrison, 1970). Further a correlation has been found between the lethal effect of ordinary unlabelled Synkavit on clone cultures and its uptake as shown by the tritium labelled compound (Dendy, 1970).

The biochemical aspects of the mechanisms of action of Synkavit have been reviewed by Mitchell and Marrian (1965). Marrian (1959) found that Synkavit reduces the uptake of labelled formate or glycine into the purines of RNA in EAT cells (see also Gronow, 1963). Chipperfield and Marrian (1962) found that Synkavit reduces the ATP content of EAT cells both *in vitro* and *in vivo*. Harrison (1968) has shown that, in EAT cells *in vitro*, 10^{-5} M Synkavit reduces the incorporation of labelled ribonucleosides and thymidine into RNA and DNA respectively, and into the acid soluble nucleotide pool, with concomitant release into the medium of the corresponding nucleoside or its degradation products. 'These effects are only observed fully when the pH of the medium is greater than 7·0 and when it contains glucose, but they are not dependent on oxygen'. Probably one of the most important effects of Synkavit acting through menadione is to reduce the synthesis and amount of ATP in the cell. The biochemical effects of menadione as a non-phosphorylative shunt by uncoupling oxidative phosphorylation, and by oxidation of NADH and NADPH, inhibition of aerobic glycolysis and stimulation of the pentose shunt pathway of glucose metabolism have been discussed by Mitchell and Marrian, 1965; see also Gordon, Ernster and Dallner, 1967; Görög and Kovács, 1967; Kupfer and Peets, 1968; Galeotti, Azzi and Chance, 1970). Of great interest is the finding of radiosensitisation by Synkavit of the loss of intracellular K^+ ions from Ehrlich ascites carcinoma cells following irradiation with 15 MeV electrons and X-rays (Flemming, Mehrishi and Napier, 1968). In connection with the problem of the relative deficiency of ubiquinones in some malignant tumours (Wattenberg, 1961; Osterberg and Wattenberg, 1961; Sugimura, Okabe and Baba, 1962; Chipperfield, 1966; but see also Tranzer and Pearse, 1963), it must be mentioned that Chipperfield (1966) found an increase in the concentration of ubiquinones on a wet weight basis in some human tumours, although on the basis of concentration per mg DNA, there was a statistically significant average decrease of 36 %, except in the case of a carcinoma of the pancreas. Further study of this subject is desirable. It was found by Birdsall (1967) that there was no evidence of selective uptake of either tritiated ubiquinol-9 or tritiated ubiquinol-0 in the Walker rat carcinosarcoma 256 after intravenous injection.

It is likely that menadione is the active form of Synkavit in the radiosensitisation of tumours. It is interesting that it also appears to be the active form of vitamin K5 (Synkamin, 2-methyl-4-amino-1-naphthol hydrochloride) in the process of radiosensitisation of various micro-organisms, studied by a group at the Massachusetts Institute of Technology in connection with the preservation of foods by irradiation (Shehata, 1961; Silverman, Shehata and Goldblith, 1962; Silverman, 1963; Bridges, 1969; see also Singh, Shenoy and Gopal-Ayengar, 1970). It is well known that menadione reacts with many -SH compounds *in vitro* (Friedmann, Marrian and Simon-Reuss, 1948). It may be mentioned that Slater (1966, 1967) found that DNA polymerase (E.C. 2.7.7.7.), prepared from mouse Ehrlich ascites tumour cells, is inhibited *in vitro* by menadione, in addition to a number of other -SH reagents, and also by Synkavit itself and to a lesser but significant extent by the dimethyl analogue, 2,3-dimethyl-1,4-naphthaquinol-bis(disodium phosphate), our compound 28; further studies of these and related phosphorylated compounds would be of interest. It may be noted that the -SH group of the DNA-polymerase molecule is probably not part of the active site (Kornberg, 1969).

For a long time I thought that 'selective radiosensitisation of the tumour cells by Compound I (Synkavit) may be envisaged as the converse of -SH protection against ionizing radiation' (Mitchell, 1960, p. 117). However, since the work of Adams (1967, 1968) and Adams and Cooke (1969) on 'electron-affinic radiosensitisation' much further clarification of the role of -SH groups is needed both from the point of view of the actions of Synkavit and more generally in relation to the mechanisms of the biological actions of ionizing radiations. The classical work of Eldjarn and Pihl (1960) suggested that only a small proportion of the total -SH groups in a cell is involved in the initial lesions produced by radiation. It is of interest to refer to the studies of this problem, using Ehrlich ascites tumour cells treated *in vivo* with tritium-labelled MNDP, carried out here by Gronow (1966). It was found that in relation to the unirradiated, between one-third and one-half of the protein-bound activity of the isolated cells was released within a few minutes after irradiation of the mice with a dose of 1,000 rads of 14 MeV X-rays delivered in one minute by means of the linear accelerator. These findings appear to provide evidence that a radiosensitive process in the tumour cells is associated with particular thiol groups.

It seems to me that the critical thiol groups may anchor the menadione formed, or some other closely related metabolite of Synkavit, in proximity to the molecule of the radiosensitive target, which is probably DNA. Menadione does not appear to form intercalation complexes with DNA, in the way that, e.g. certain acridines are intercalated between the base pairs of DNA (Lerman, 1961; Neville and Davies, 1966). It is of interest that following the electron spin resonance studies of Nicolau, Körner and Cristea (1966, 1967), Mr T. Morley has found that not only menadione but also S-(2-methyl-1,4-naphthaquinonyl-3-)glutathione, 'thiodione', increased by a factor of about 1·4, the yield of free radicals produced by irradiation of DNA in freeze-dried molecular mixtures with the quinones, in relation to DNA alone. Thus the presence of the S-glutathionyl group in the 3-position on menadione does not affect the increase in the total radical yield. It is clear that in these experiments, menadione and a number of related quinones are very effective electron acceptors.

(ii) *The possibilities of radioactive drugs*

It seems to me to be important at the present time to try to develop radioactive drugs which are concentrated selectively in the viable malignant cells of tumours and carry incorporated radioactive atoms in sufficiently high specific activity to the right place in the tumour, and in the malignant cells in order to produce the necessary radiotherapeutic effect *in situ*, without significant damage to the normal tissues. I have envisaged this as a new approach to the chemotherapy of cancer and called it 'radio-chemotherapy' (Mitchell, 1968).

A large number of labelled compounds have been described in the literature as 'tumour seekers' (Mitchell, 1969, 1970). Some of these have proved to be useful in the clinical diagnosis and localisation of malignant tumours, mainly by means of scintigraphy. However, in general, these compounds do not show a sufficiently high degree of selective concentration in the tumour in relation to the critical normal tissues to be applicable in therapy. So far, no labelled compound is known, which has a degree of selective concentration in tumours comparable with that of iodine in the normal thyroid gland. Moreover, the present trend in tracer studies is to use short-lived isotopes in order to reduce the radiation doses to the normal tissues.

The development of radioactive drugs for therapeutic purposes presents many difficulties. The choice of the chemical compound to serve as the carrier of the radioactive isotope is, of course, the central problem. Another difficulty which emerges with the study of radioactive drugs but which is also encountered in the chemotherapy of solid tumours is the frequent inaccessibility to the drugs, of parts of tumours, which nevertheless contain viable malignant cells, because of defective blood supply. As confirmed by angiography, this is especially the case with large masses of tumour. However, it seems to me that it is possible that a radioactive drug could be curative, since ionizing radiations are the only agents apart from surgery, which as yet have cured substantial numbers of patients with cancer.

SELECTION OF THE RADIONUCLIDE FOR INCORPORATION INTO A RADIOACTIVE DRUG

At the present time, most of the studies of possible radioactive drugs have concerned uses of the two isotopes, radioactive hydrogen, Tritium (^{3}H) (Mitchell, 1965a, b, 1966, 1967a, b, 1968, 1969, 1970) and the radio-iodine isotope, ^{131}I. As is well known, since 1942 radio-iodine has been used in inorganic form in the treatment of carcinoma of the thyroid (Keston *et al.*, 1942; Seidlin *et al.*, 1949). Radio-iodine therapy appears to be useful as a model for the development of radioactive drugs, but in making this point, one must note its limitations.

It is reasonable to study suitable organic compounds incorporating ^{131}I in high specific activity. For example, the experience we have gained recently in clinical uptake studies with 6-^{131}I-iodo-MNDP, with preparations of specific activity up to about 2 mCi per mg suggests the possibility of investigations from the point of view of therapy with preparations of considerably higher specific activity. However, much further work with ^{131}I is necessary. The application of ^{124}I is possible but not very hopeful from the point of view of developing organic compounds as radioactive drugs for therapy (Phillips, 1957; Phillips, Haybittle and Newbery, 1960).

Tritium (^{3}H) appears to be very suitable for this investigation, or at least for elucidation of the problems. Its radiobiological action is localised in single cells or cell constituents. It is a pure beta-ray emitter, with very soft beta-radiation, with a maximum range of about 6 μm in water and soft tissue of unit density. The mean energy of the beta particles is $5{\cdot}73 \pm 0{\cdot}03$ keV and the corresponding range in unit density tissue is approximately 0·9 μm. The radioactive half-life is 12·4 years but almost invariably the values of the biological half-life observed for human tissues and tumours with the radioactive drugs studied have been very much less, often between 3 and 14 days. For uniformly distributed tritium at a stationary concentration, 1 mCi per g of tissue delivers a dose rate of 293 rads per day.

It is of some importance that the introduction of tritium as a hydrogen isotope into an organic molecule causes no change in its chemical structure or pharmacological properties. Moreover, the handling of a number of relevant tritiated compounds presents no really serious difficulties in therapeutic applications.

The use of isotopes of some other elements in soluble organic form has been suggested, e.g. arsenic (Lettré, 1946), for which ^{74}As of half-life 18 days is the most suitable isotope, and mercury (Ganatra, 1969 – personal communication), using the isotope ^{203}Hg of half-life 47 days. It would be interesting to use an isotope emitting α-particles; this might be possible experimentally using astatine, At^{211}, of half-life 7·3 hours, which behaves rather like iodine and in inorganic form concentrates in the thyroid galnd (Hamilton, 1942; Hamilton *et al.*, 1956). Radio-carbon, ^{14}C, is not suitable for therapeutic applications, primarily because of its long half-life of 5,760 years.

SOME QUANTITATIVE CONSIDERATIONS

In thinking quantitatively about this problem, it is useful to start with the Differential Absorption Ratio (D.A.R.) defined as the ratio of specific activity of the tumour – or relevant normal tissue – to the mean specific activity of the body as a whole.

As a basis for the calculation of the radiation dose delivered by a particular isotope, one must obviously have detailed information not only about the decay scheme and physical half-life of the isotope but also about the specific activity of the isotope in the tumour and in the normal tissues and the corresponding values of the biological half-life, or preferably the related mean life, as an expression of the average time which the isotope stays in the cells. The relevant 'critical organs' are in most cases, bone marrow and lymphoid tissue, kidneys and gonads – sometimes liver, gastro-intestinal tract, bones, thyroid or eyes. It is important to note that experience of the treatment of carcinoma of the thyroid with radio-iodine, ^{131}I, has shown that there is no evidence of long-term damage to the kidney (Pochin, 1969).

As a first approximation, it is reasonable to assume a uniform distribution of the radioactivity both in the tumour and at a much lower level in the body as a whole. In this case, evidence can be deduced from the experience of radiotherapy with external beams. If one treated a small squamous carcinoma of the skin with a single dose of ^{60}Co or ^{137}Cs gamma-rays at high dose rate (with suitable build-up), one would need a minimum tumour dose of at least 2,100 rads and perhaps up to 3,000 rads. In whole body irradiation with external γ-ray sources, the critical organ at the lower dose levels is the bone marrow, as is likely to be the case with many radioactive drugs. The cancer patients tend to be frail, so that the maximum single dose of the same radiation that could be given safely to the whole body at high dose rate, without producing serious early or late damage, can be estimated at 150 rads, though in some cases it might be wise not to exceed about 75 rads. If these doses were delivered at high dose rates by a radioactive substance accumulating in the tumour tissue, with a uniform distribution, and with a concentration in the bone marrow equal to the average throughout the rest of the body, the DAR in the tumour would need to be at least 14 to 20 and preferably about 30 to 40.

In fact, of course, the radiation is usually delivered by the radioactive drugs at relatively low dose rates. It turns out that in the most favourable cases, the biological half-life, is substanially less for the critical normal tissues, and for the whole body, than for the malignant tumour. Moreover, one appears to gain a real advantage by repeated injections of the radioactive drugs. It seems possible that in this way, the DAR necessary for therapy could be reduced considerably, even to values as low as about 4 to 8 in some circumstances. Nevertheless, for the assumption of uniform distribution of the radioactivity in the tumour, it would seem to be wise to aim at a value of the DAR of at least about 15 to 20 and preferably at least about 30.

As the next step, it is useful to consider the problem of radio-iodine therapy of carcinoma of the thyroid using ^{131}I. It may be of interest to refer briefly to a patient of mine. He was a 26-year old road worker with an inoperable carcinoma of the thyroid with extensive lymph-node metastases – the histology being large celled follicular adenocarcinoma of the thyroid. The tumour became operable after radio-iodine (^{131}I) therapy and after the operation further radio-iodine therapy was given. The patient is still well after 17 years. The mean value of the initial DAR for a large metastasis in a lymph node was found to be 31, while the value for the primary tumour was 131 (Phillips, 1954, 1955).

Further consideration is necessary to take into account the inhomogeneity of the distribution of the isotope observed in many tumours, both primary and secondary. For example of ^{131}I in inorganic form, autoradiographs have shown that in a typical case of thyroid carcinoma which concentrates radio-iodine, the uptake of iodine is grossly non-uniform with inactive gaps often of dimensions 1 to 5 mm. The maximum range of the β-rays is only 2 mm and the dose contribution from the γ-rays is usually small, so that there are regions of tumour which receive practically no radiation. This has been confirmed histologically (e.g. Phillips, 1954). This difficulty should be largely overcome by the use of the alternative isotope ^{124}I (Phillips, 1957; Phillips, Haybittle and Newbery, 1960); unfortunately, it has only been possible to use this isotope in the treatment of a very few patients, because its production by the reaction ^{121}Sb (α,n) ^{124}I requires a cyclotron and is apparently rather difficult.

For a particular isotope of known physical properties, it is often possible to deduce an approximate value of the mean tumour cell dose. As will be seen, this appears to be useful from a clinical point of view, even though the value of the minimum tumour cell dose may be the factor limiting curability. The most direct method of doing this is by the investigation of biopsy, surgical or autopsy specimens by means of histological and autoradiographic studies, in conjunction with measurements of the specific activity of the isotope in the tissue specimen. In many tumours, there is an important component, consisting of stroma and necrotic areas and also acini in some cases of adenocarcinoma, which have only very low uptake of the radioactive drug. Usually the malignant cells showing uptake – which appear at least superficially to be the viable cells – occupy at most one half of the total volume of the tumour mass and often a much smaller proportion, e.g. from one-third to one-sixth. This proportion varies greatly in different parts of the primary and secondary tumours, and from a practical point of view can only be evaluated on relatively small samples.

As we shall consider for the example of Synkavit, clinical radioisotope scanning with ^{131}I-labelled compounds is being studied as a rapid method for determining the selective concentration of the compound and its distribution in the tumour and normal tissues in the individual patient. By means of measurements on a 'phantom' model of the tumour containing the isotope with a uniform distribution, the mean value of the DAR can be determined approximately. With the scanning techniques used, this value represents an average over inhomogeneities of concentration of dimensions up to a few millimetres. Accordingly, if the malignant cells responsible for the uptake occupy, e.g. $\frac{1}{2}$ to $\frac{1}{3}$ of the total volume of the tumour, the mean DAR in the malignant cells could be higher by a factor of 2 to 3 than the mean calculated for a uniform distribution; in particular, a small correction has to be made for the low level of uptake in the stroma, necrotic areas and acini. These considerations lead to the provisional conclusion that the DAR, measured in the usual was by quantitative scanning procedures in conjunction with phantom studies, should in general reach a macroscopic average value of at least about 7 to be useful in therapeutic applications. Higher values are obviously desirable. Much further work is necessary in this field.

THE CHOICE OF COMPOUND: THE KEY QUESTION

A quite surprising number of compounds have been investigated. I have summarised these elsewhere (Mitchell, 1969, 1970). In our present approach to this problem, we are going back to Paul Ehrlich's aphorism '*Corpora non agunt, nisi fixata*'.

A long time ago in 1911, Wassermann *et al.* observed that certain dyes are concentrated in tumour tissue. The first really relevant experiments were those of Kottmann (1935) in Bern, showing the striking affinity for tumours of certain iodine-containing substituted naphthalene-sulphonic acids. With some of these compounds, especially 1-iodo-8-naphthol-3,6-disulphonic acid, he observed radiosensitisation of transplanted tumours in mice with X-rays. Arising out of this work, were the important investigations of ^{82}Br labelled derivatives, in particular ^{82}Br labelled 1-amino-8-naphthol-3,6-disulphonate by Kroll, Strauss and Necheles (1941) and later the practical application of di-^{131}I-iodo-fluorescein by Moore (1948) in the diagnosis of cerebral tumours.

Clinical investigations have been carried out with many compounds, mainly since the introduction of scintigraphy. However, only a few of these have been studied clinically from a therapeutic point of view and the evidence about these may be summarised before discussing our work with tritiated MNDP, as follows:

(i) *Rose Bengal incorporating* ^{131}I

This dye which is a fluorescein derivative, incorporating ^{131}I was used in doses of up to 65 mCi by Ariel and Pack (1960) in an attempt to obtain palliative treatment in cases of carcinoma of the biliary passages. Recently, Shoop (1969) found that the labelled dye was concentrated in a functional hepatoma.

(ii) *Antibodies to fibrin and fibrinogen, incorporating* ^{131}I

It has been known for a long time that extra-vascular deposits of fibrin are found in malignant tumours. Day, Planinsek and Pressman (1959) were able to show that antibodies to rat fibrin labelled with ^{131}I had a clear-cut affinity for some transplanted rat tumours. Since then, this approach has led to interesting results, e.g. Spar *et al.* (1967) obtained palliative results in the treatment of 12 patients with advanced malignant tumours of various types with intravenous injections of anti-human fibrinogen antibodies incorporating ^{131}I with doses of 100–160 mCi, together with subsequent treatment with Epsilon-aminocaproic acid as an antifibrinolytic agent.

(iii) *Tritiated thymidine of high specific activity, e.g. up to 20 Ci/mM*

Everyone knows that tritium-labelled thymidine is incorporated into the DNA of proliferating cells. There is, however, no appreciable selective uptake into tumour cells. The concentration process depends on the partial pressure of oxygen in the tumour tissue (Rajewsky, 1965). The prospects for the use of tritiated thymidine in clinical treatment are not encouraging, particularly in view of the practical difficulties in handling large amounts of tritiated thymidine of high specific activity.

(iv) *Tritiated derivatives of MNDP (Synkavit) of the highest possible specific activity, and some related compounds*

This is the work of a team in Cambridge since 1953. Qualitative information about the distribution of Synkavit and some related compounds in the rat in different organs, with evidence of concentration in the Walker carcinosarcoma 256, especially in the growing edge of the tumour, had been obtained by studies of the fluorescence with Wood's light of derivatives produced by treatment of the cut surfaces of tissues with alkaline hydrogen peroxide (Mitchell, 1949, 1953, 1955). The limitations of fluorescence methods were recognised and more precise studies were then made using compounds with radioactive labelling.

In this way, by means of labelling of MNDP (Synkavit) and some related compounds, with C^{14}, Br^{82}, I^{131} and finally tritium, we were able to show selective concentration in certain experimental tumours in animals and in some human tumours (Maxwell, 1954, 1955; Marrian and Maxwell, 1956a, b; Marrian, 1957; Horwitz *et al.*, 1959). The first tritiated preparations T1, used in 1959 were made by the Wilzbach procedure but these unfortunately contained tritiated water as an impurity, which was toxic to the bone marrow in certain cases. However, since September 1960 all the tritiated preparations have been made by chemical synthesis, the tritium being incorporated by means of catalytic dehydrogenation of the corresponding halogen derivatives (Andrews *et al.*, 1962). The tritium is present in stable positions in the molecule. This work is a joint effort of the Department of Radiotherapeutics, University of Cambridge, the Radiochemical Centre, Amersham, Bucks., and Roche Products, Welwyn Garden City. We have used three main preparations described according to the catalogue of the Radiochemical Centre as TRA 72, containing one atom of tritium per molecule in the 6-position, TRA 119 which in theory contained 3 atoms of tritium per molecule in the 5, 6 and 7-positions and finally TRK 219, which is the most reliable so far (see Fig. 2). TRK 219 is 2-methyl-6,7-ditritio-1,4-naphthaquinol-bis(disodium phosphate). It contains two tritium atoms per molecule, with theoretical specific activity 58·2 Ci per mmol, and one Ci is contained in 7·3 mg of chemical. An attempt is being made to prepare the compound with 4 tritium atoms per molecule (Hodgson, 1968; Thomas, 1970).

With these radioactive drugs, one needs a higher degree of radiopharmaceutical purity – as well as radiochemical purity – than has been thought necessary previously. Even now, the

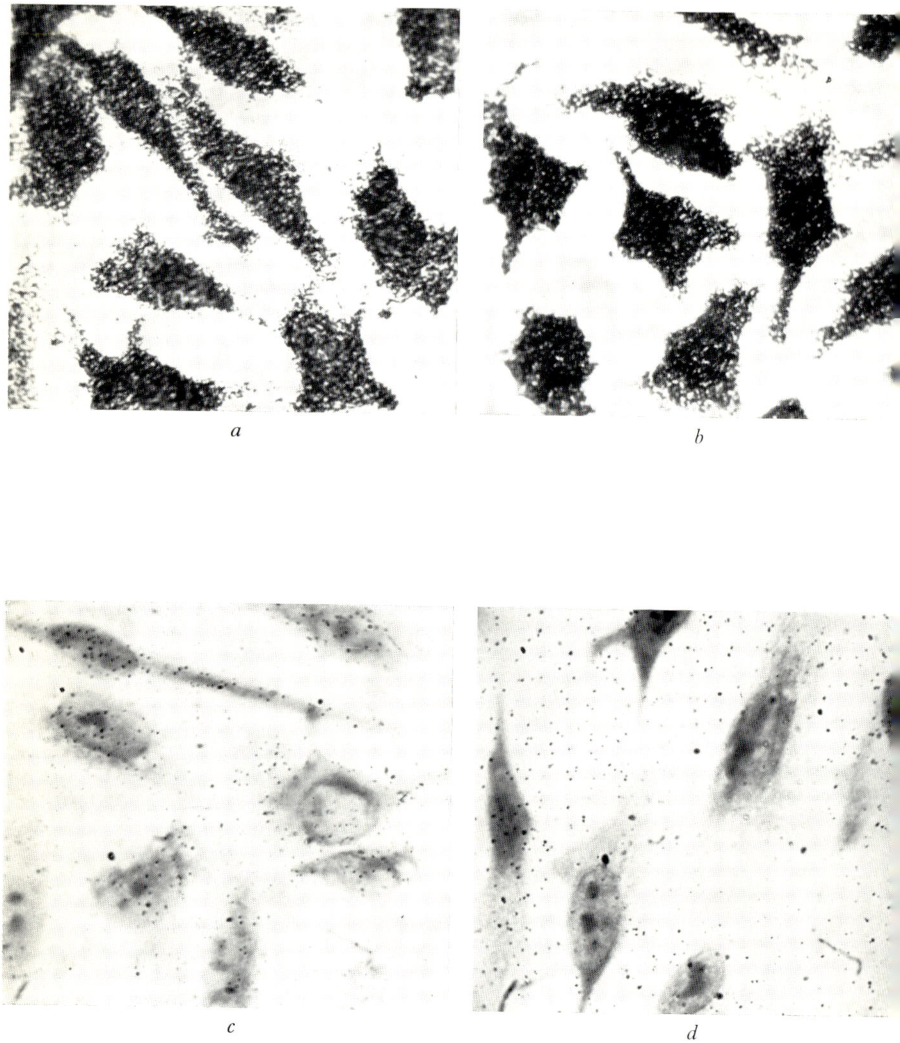

Fig. 3 Autoradiographs of batch 109 of the tritiated drug, TRK 219, acceptable for clinical use:

(*a*) HEp/2 cells.
(*b*) HeLa cells.
(*c*) Fresh monkey kidney cells.
(*d*) Fresh human amnion cells.

(For detail of technique, see Dendy, 1969.)

individual batches of TRK 219 may differ in their biological properties. For this reason, we still test them on tissue cultures with autoradiography to be certain of a high degree of selective uptake into cells of tumour strains (HeLa and Hep 2) with negligible uptake into cells of normal origin, e.g. human amnion epithelium, and also human embryonal skin and lung epithelium, together with monkey kidney cells (Simon-Reuss, 1961; Dendy, 1969). A 'bad' batch may show uptake into the normal cells. Quantitatively, 'good' batches show 30 times the uptake in the tumour cells as in the normal cells – sometimes even higher ratios (Fig. 3). It is now certain that some freshly cultured human tumour cells take up TRK 219 *invitro*. In the routine testing, it has emerged that the selective concentration of Synkavit and TRK 219 in the tumour cells *in vivo* only occurs within the concentration range $1{\cdot}5 \times 10^{-5}$ M to $1{\cdot}5 \times 10^{-4}$ M. Moreover, the uptake is pH depend nt, falling off rapidly below pH 7·0. We have studied this in animal experiments and the same is probably true for human tumours. This factor seems to be very important.

We have carried out systematic experiments with the radioactive drugs on rabbits to exclude both acute toxicity on intravenous injection and chronic radio-toxicity during the rest of the life span of the animal. In the earlier stages of the work, we gained a great deal of confidence from studies of the treatment of spontaneous tumours in cats and dogs by our veterinary colleague Dr I. A. Silver (see Silver *et al.*, 1962). For example, 5 out of 7 cases of carcinoma of the tongue and palate in cats responded favourably to intra-arterial injection of quite small doses of the tritiated drugs and two of these have lived longer than two years.

THE PRESENT STATE OF THE CLINICAL INVESTIGATIONS

Up to the end of July 1969, in all 174 patients with various types of advanced, recurrent, inoperable histologically verified malignant tumours and reticuloses were treated with tritiated derivatives of MNDP. These drugs were only used when all other therapeutic measures – surgery, conventional radiotherapy and chemotherapy – had failed or were definitely contra-indicated. One very useful finding at the beginning of this work was the frequent relief of pain: one of our earliest cases was able to give up morphia. This encouraged us to continue.

The clinical assessment of the results of the treatment has often proved to be difficult. I finally accepted evidence of reduction in size of tumour as an objective criterion of response, even though it is modest. I have been very strict; all doubtful results were rigorously excluded.

The clinical studies so far fall into two parts (Tables 2a and b). The first part corresponds to the exploratory phase which in the literature of cancer chemotherapy is often called the First Phase. In this investigation it overlaps to some extent with the second part.

As discussed earlier (p. 30) it was found by the use of the statistical method developed by Gehan (1961) that there was a definite effect in 16 of the first 102 cases. As an approximate method of analysing the effect of dose, the total amount of tritiated drug administered appeared to be the simplest criterion. All the patients classified as treated received a total dose of at least 1 Ci. Low doses were defined as 1–9·5 Ci administered by intra-arterial routes, or 1–19·5 Ci by the intravenous route, while high doses were defined as 10 Ci or more intra-arterially, or 20 Ci or more intravenously. The proportion of patients showing a positive response was 10 out of 23, i.e. 43·5% with the high doses but only 6 out of 79, i.e. 7·6% with the low doses. This difference is highly significant statistically ($P<0{\cdot}001$). No statistically significant difference was found between the proportion of responses after intra-arterial and intra-venous administration.

The aim of the Second Phase of the clinical investigations is to determine the indications for the application of the radioactive drugs and the right lines for their practical dosage, with special consideration of the problem of repetition ('fractionation') and timing of the injections.

Among the total number of 174 patients treated so far in both parts of the investigations, a definite reduction in size of the tumour was observed in 25, that is in 14·4% of all cases. Obviously the

Table 2(a). *Clinical assessment of the radioactive drugs First part of the investigation 1959–63*

85 patients with advanced recurrent inoperable histologically verified malignant tumours and reticuloses were treated with T1 (25 patients), TRA 72 (16 patients) and TRA 119 (44 patients) between 4 February 1959 and 12 December 1963. The numbers in brackets show the number of cases in which there was objective evidence of definite reduction in the size of the tumour.

	No. of cases	
Diagnosis	Intravenous injection	Intra-arterial administration
Adenocarcinoma of the gastro-intestinal tract:		
Carcinoma of the stomach	3 (1)	0
Carcinoma of the colon	1 (0)	4 (0)
Carcinoma of the rectum	2 (0)	6 (0)
Carcinoma of the gall bladder	1 (0)	0
Bronchial carcinoma	1 (0)	8 (0)
Malignant melanoma of skin	3 (0)	2 (1)
Glioma – incomplete surgery	0	7 (0)
Carcinoma of the breast	5 (1)	0
Carcinoma of the ovary	1 (1)	3 (0)
Carcinoma of the cervix	0	3 (1)
Carcinoma of the vagina	0	1 (1)
Tumours of the kidney		2 (0)
Bone sarcomata	2 (0)	3 (2)
Various tumours	10 (0)	9 (0)
Radiosensitive tumours and reticuloses:		
Seminoma	1 (1)	1 (1)
Hodgkin's disease	2 (1)	0
Chronic lymphatic leukaemia	1 (1)	0
Neuroblastoma	1 (0)	1 (0)
Mycosis fungoides	1 (0)	0
Total	35 (6)	50 (6)

clinical observations in the individual patients must be taken into account. Accordingly, the results of treatment have proved to be in general modest, sometimes useful, and in a few cases impressive.

Palliative effects were observed in certain selected patients with advanced inoperable malignant tumours and reticuloses of the following types: carcinoma of the stomach and colon, carcinoma of the gall bladder, malignant melanoma of the skin, carcinoma of the ovary, bone sarcomata – (though only with intra-arterial administration) – seminoma and Hodgkin's disease. Our recent results suggest that carcinoma of the pancreas should be investigated further.

Relief of pain was estimated by a clear-cut reduction of the doses of analgesic agents required, including morphia. Twenty-four patients showed definite relief of pain. In addition, in one case of Hodgkin's disease, the intense generalised pruritus disappeared within four hours after an intravenous injection of three curies of TRA 119.

It is of interest to consider the results with TRK 219 in further detail. Among the 78 patients with advanced disease treated with intravenous TRK 219 (see Table 2b), palliative results were obtained in 1 out of 8 cases of carcinoma of the stomach, 3 out of 15 cases of carcinoma of the colon, one case of carcinoma of the gall bladder, 3 out of 11 cases of malignant melanoma of the skin and 1 out of 3 cases of carcinoma of the ovary. Among the selected cases of the radiosensitive neoplastic conditions, the one patient with testicular seminoma, a man of 31 with pulmonary metastases initially, treated with TRK 219 pre-operatively, though requiring external radiotherapy, has survived 4 years 9 months with minimal symptoms and the one patient with Hodgkin's disease, a man of 20, has survived well and free from symptoms 5 years after TRK 219 treatment of a histologically verified recurrence in cervical lymph nodes which previously had been heavily irradiated. Too great an importance should not be attached to either of these cases.

Most of the results have only been palliative though sometimes very useful.

In one remarkable advanced case of mucinous cystadenocarcinoma of the ovary, there was autoradiographic evidence of

Table 2(b). *Clinical assessment of the radiactive drugs (cont.)*
Second part of the investigation 1964–69

89 patients with advanced recurrent inoperable histologically verified malignant tumours and reticuloses were treated with TRK 219 between 24 September 1964 and 23 July 1969. The numbers in brackets show the number of cases in which there was objective evidence of definite reduction in the size of the tumour.

Diagnosis	No. of cases Intravenous injection	 Intra-arterial administration
Adenocarcinoma of the gastro-intestinal tract:		
Carcinoma of the stomach	8 (1)	0
Carcinoma of the colon	15 (3)	0
Carcinoma of the rectum	6 (0)	1 (0)
Carcinoma of the gall bladder	1 (1)	0
Bronchial carcinoma	4 (0)	0
Malignant melanoma of skin	11 (3)	1 (1)
Glioma – incomplete surgery	0	5 (0)
Carcinoma of the breast	4 (0)	0
Carcinoma of the ovary	3 (1)	0
Carcinoma of the cervix	2 (0)	1 (0)
Tumours of the kidney	3 (0)	1 (0)
Bone sarcomata	4 (0)	0
Various tumours	14 (0)	2 (1*)
Radiosensitive tumours and reticuloses:		
Seminoma	1 (1[a])	0
Hodgkin's disease	1 (1[b])	0
Mycosis fungoides	1 (0)	0
Total	78 (11)	11 (2)

[a] Surviving 4 years 9 months. [b] Surviving 5 years without symptoms.
* Carcinoma of antrum.

selective uptake of TRK 219 into a group of cells regarded at tumour cells in the sternal bone marrow, in a smear taken at 32 minutes after intravenous injection of 3·2 Ci in 28 mg of compound.

The patient, a lady of 58, had had an operation for carcinoma of the ovary, with post-operative radiotherapy, in the previous year. She was admitted for terminal care in a very poor general condition with widespread metastases in the bones of the skull and pelvis and in the lungs with bilateral pleural effusions after no response to chlorambucil and prednisone. She was treated by means of a course of intravenous injections of TRK 219 and received a total amount of 28·6 Ci in 9 injections in 29 days. Prednisone 10 mg daily was continued. After being rather ill, though relieved by aspiration of the right pleural effusion and a transfusion, she improved considerably in general condition and the palpable tumour masses became less tender and slightly smaller. She got up again and put on weight; in fact she acquired a new flat and bought new furniture and also went away for a holiday. She had three months of almost normal activity but then deteriorated with increasing size of the tumour masses, though with an essentially normal blood count, and died six weeks later. The autopsy showed carcinomatosis.

Of some interest is a patient, a lady of 40, who was also a diabetic treated with Tolbutamide, who had numerous metastases of malignant melanoma on the stump and inguinal region after an amputation through the left thigh, chemotherapy with Melphalan and radiotherapy. The most recent radiotherapy consisted of four treatments each of maximum dose 300 rad of 15 MeV X-rays delivered between 8 and 4 days before the first intravenous injection of 8·7 Ci of TRK 219 in 65 mg of Compound. During the 5 weeks, after this injection, many metastatic nodules first became darkly pigmented and then fell off as black crusts, leaving depigmented skin areas. Other skin metastases gradually disappeared although despite two further injections of TRK 219, new metastases became obvious and grew. The new metastases appeared first on the outer side of the thigh in an area which had not been included in the most recent X-ray field. It may be suggested that the relatively small dose of radiation given during the 8 days before the first TRK 219 injection led to increased vascularity of the metastases in the treated area, and perhaps also to reduced lactic acid concentration and possibly to increased synthesis of alkaline phosphatase, with resulting high uptake of the TRK 219 into the tumour cells of this area. In association with the local improvement, there was a striking subjective improvement in the patient's general condition but unfortunately after two months, the patient died with extensive metastases.

A clinical problem which has arisen is the occurrence of necrosis in tumour masses within the body after treatment with the radioactive drugs. This leads to toxic absorption and a clinical picture similar to 'crush syndrome', and requires similar treatment. Striking examples of this problem were seen in a case of advanced carcinoma of the gall bladder, where the toxic absorption was probably the cause of death, and in a case of advanced carcinoma of the pancreas.

The 'Third Phase' of this development now in progress is the treatment of selected patients with clearly defined indications, including evidence of selective uptake of MNDP into the tumour. At the same time we are trying to increase the selective uptake of the radioactive drugs into the tumour cells, e.g. by pre-treatment with oral sodium or potassium citrate mixture and/or fasting overnight before each injection. Pre-treatment with hyperbaric oxygen does not appear hopeful but must be investigated further.

SCANNING WITH ^{131}I LABELLED COMPOUNDS

In order to develop a practical method for rapid determination of the selective concentration of MNDP and its distribution in the in tumour individual cases, the ^{131}I labelled compound, 6-^{131}I-iodo-MNDP, was prepared and its uptake has been studied so far (to 11.4.1970) in 51 patients with advanced tumours by means of radio-isotope scanning (Marrian *et al.*, 1969; Mitchell, 1969, 1970). Positive results have been obtained in certain cases of carcinoma of the colon, stomach and pancreas and in one case of advanced tubular adenocarcinoma of the kidney.

A particularly striking example is shown in Fig. 4 for an advanced case of carcinoma of the pancreas. The uptake of the 6-^{131}I-iodo-MNDP appears to correspond closely with the distribution of the tumour found at operation; in addition, there is excretion into the gall bladder. In this case, the interpretation of the scan is unambiguous except for the detailed distribution of the activity in relation to the metastases in the liver. Subsequently antero-posterior and lateral scans were used to deduce the size and position of the primary tumour mass; its volume was estimated at approximately 400 ml. From measurements on a phantom model, it was calculated that the value of the macroscopic average DAR for the uptake of the compound into the primary tumour mass was 6 to 8, say 7. From measurements of a histological section of the biopsy specimen, it was found that the tumour cells occupied about one-fifth of the volume of the piece of tissue studied; hence, the value of the DAR for the tumour cells in at least some areas was possibly about 35.

The correspondence between the distribution of activity observed in the scans and the known distribution of viable tumour was, in general, close but certain discrepancies, which are difficult to understand, have been encountered. It has been shown that the evidence concerning uptake into tumours obtained using 6-^{131}I-iodo-MNDP and tritiated MNDP (TRK 219) can be complementary (see Fig. 2); it is possible that the biological half-lives are shorter for the former than for the latter compound. In all but the earliest scans, the picture may be confused by excretion by the liver into the bile; there is usually accumulation in the gall-bladder, with subsequent concentration in the colon. In some cases, it is difficult to distinguish uptake in metastases in the liver from the presence of the labelled compound in normal liver tissue; supple-

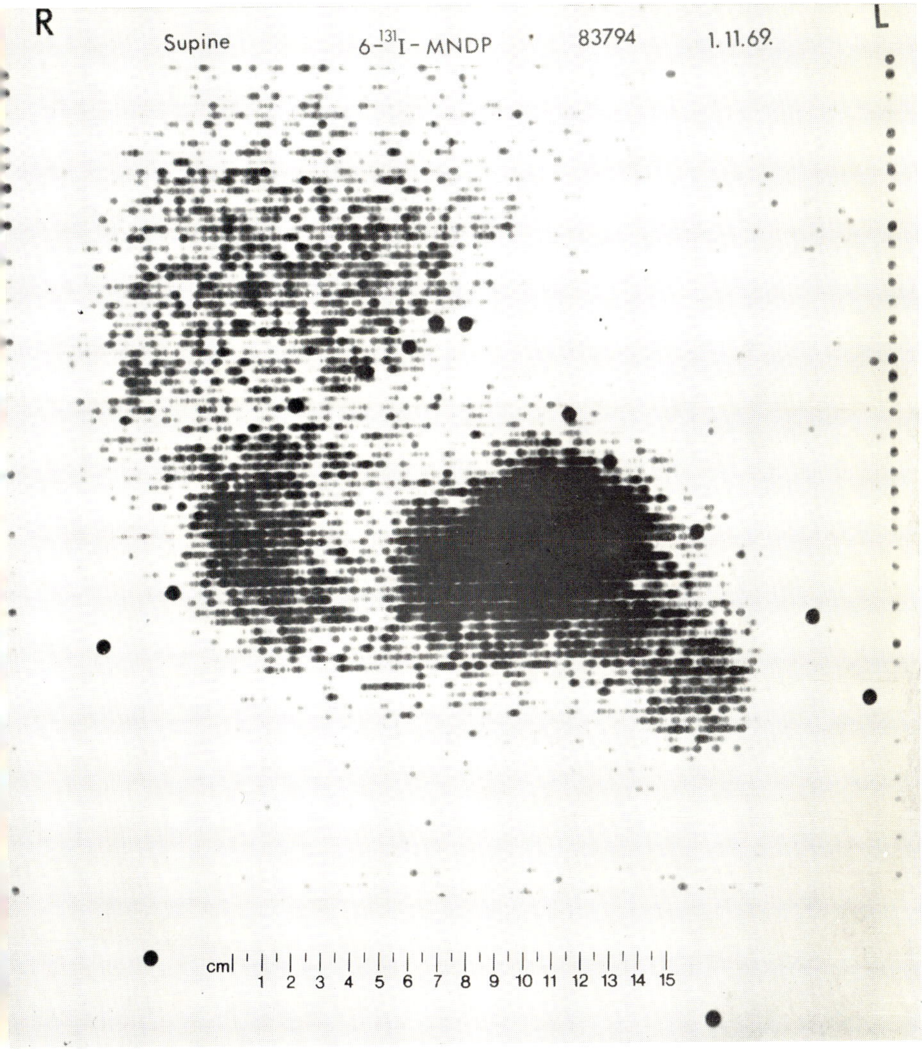

Fig. 4 Photoscan at 23 to 67 minutes after intravenous injection of 460 μCi in 12·5 mg 6-^{131}I-iodo-MNDP in a patient, a man of 52, with an inoperable histologically verified carcinoma of the tail of the pancreas, involving the transverse colon and stomach and with retroperitoneal extension downwards and laterally together with multiple metastases in the liver.

The uptake of the 6-^{131}I-iodo-MNDP appears to correspond closely with the distribution of the tumour found at operation; in addition, there is excretion by the normal liver tissue and accumulation in the gall bladder.

mentary evidence can be obtained by scanning with ^{99m}Tc sulphur colloid. At present, to try to clarify this problem, an attempt is being made to determine the optimal specific activity of the 6-^{131}I-iodo-MNDP for scanning. In any case, it is important to follow the course of the uptake with time and probably to scan at the time of maximum accumulation in the tumour. Recently, the activity injected has varied between 400 and 1,000 μCi. These activities are regarded as acceptable in the investigation of the individual patients under consideration; in a test using 500 μCi, the total dose of radiation to the kidneys is not likely to exceed about 2·3 rads and the dose to other normal tissues is considerably less.

It must be emphasised that much further work is required including a survey of different types of tumours, together with a detailed study of cases of adenocarcinoma of the gastro-intestinal tract, including the pancreas and particularly of early cases. It is by no means certain how far scanning with 6-^{131}I-iodo-MNDP is likely to be of general value in the diagnosis of malignant tumours. Much more evidence is required but it appears already that there is wide variation in the uptake among different malignant tumours of apparently similar type and similar histology.

Our present work with this compound was greatly influenced by the report of the research group in Bombay led by Dr R. D. Ganatra (Ganatra *et al.*, 1966). More recently he and his colleagues (Ganatra *et al.*, 1968, 1969) have published full reports on animal experiments and clinical observations with tumour scientigraphy using not only a different radio-iodine labelled Synkavit but also a labelled derivative of 6-hydroxy-2-methyl-1,4-naphthaquinone which they called 'radio-iodinated Synkol'.

PROBLEMS INVOLVED IN THE PRACTICAL DOSAGE OF THE TRITIATED DRUGS

We will now turn briefly to the difficult problem of the practical dosage in the therapeutic application of the tritiated drugs. This involves many physical and biological problems, which as yet are not completely solved.

There is extensive evidence from measurements of the specific activity of biopsy, surgical and autopsy specimens of tissues and tumours and from associated autoradiographic studies that the tritiated drugs show selective concentration in the malignant cells of certain human tumours, but very little uptake into many normal cells, including the normal cells of the bone marrow.

The measured values of the specific activity in the tumour and tissue samples must always be referred to the dose administered and to the interval of time after the injections. May I recall that for a homogeneous constant distribution, one millicurie of tritium per gram of wet tissue delivers a dose rate of 293 rads per day. This approximation is very useful, even though there is in general considerable inhomogeneity in the microscopic distribution of the tritium. The radiation dose per disintegration of tritium can be calculated for microscopic volumes (Strauss, 1958; Goodheart, 1961; Künkel, 1962; Bleecken, 1964; Stewart 1964; Tägder and Scheuermann, 1970). However, the difficult problems of realistic approximation to the exact dosimetry of the tritium of the radioactive drugs under consideration are largely unsolved. It appears to be useful to make approximate calculations of the specific activity of the tritium in the tumour cells with the help of investigations of the histology and autoradiography.

Patients appear to vary greatly in their response to the radioactive drugs. Distribution and excretion studies have shown great differences between individual patients and great variations in the values of the biological half-life of the tritium in different tumours and in normal tissues (Chipperfield, 1967a and b). 'Most of the tritiated material is excreted in the urine, a very small percentage appears in the breath as tritiated water and an even smaller percentage appears in the faeces in the first three days'. Excretion from the body by all routes in the first 3 days was measured for 14 patients; there was more than 25% excretion in all cases, 50% or more in 9 cases, and over 90% in 6 cases. For the urinary excretion, during the first 24 hours, most of the tritium was present as menadiol glycuronide, with small amounts of menadiol sulphate, menadione, another conjugate of menadione or 1,4-naphthaquinone and unchanged MNDP; after the first 24 hours, the urinary excretion products were only MNDP and the conjugate of menadione or 1,4-naphthaquinone'. Following intravenous injection of tritiated MNDP, tritiated Menaquinone-4 (Vitamin $K_2/20$) can be detected in the circulating blood after 20 minutes (Ritzl, 1968); there is also evidence of excretion of tritiated material in the bile.

With regard to the human tumours studied (Chipperfield, 1967a), the initial uptake observed in biopsy and surgical specimens taken 30 minutes after intravenous or intra-arterial injection was highest in cases of carcinoma of the gastro-intestinal tract, with values of $22{\cdot}1 \pm 8{\cdot}4$ μCi per g wet weight per Ci injected for TRK 219 and $27{\cdot}4 \pm 2{\cdot}2$ μCi per g per Ci injected for TRA 119. In some of these tumours and their metastases, there was abundant stroma with low uptake, so that the mean specific activity of the tumour cells may be considerably higher than the average value for the macroscopic specimen, e.g. in one case by a factor of 6·3. There is often wide variation among the tumour cells and different parts of the tumour. Taking into account this distribution of activity, it is possible to calculate an approximate value of the *mean tumour cell* dose, but difficult to estimate the minimum tumour cell dose, even though the uptake is limited to viable tumour cells. In a typical example of carcinoma of the colon, the specific activity of the gross specimen may be 20 μCi per g per Ci injected, so that allowing for stroma and necrotic areas by means of a factor of 3·5, the mean specific activity of the tumour cells would be 70 μCi per g per Ci and for 10 Ci injected 0·70 mCi per g; the corresponding initial mean tumour cells dose would be 205 rads per 24 hours. For a typical value of the biological half-life of 10 days and mean life 14·4 days, the total mean cell dose delivered would be 2,960, say 3,000 rads. The RBE of the tritium β-particles depends on dose rate (Hall, Oliver and Bedford, 1967).

In the present example, it seems reasonable to assume an average value of the RBE in relation to γ-rays of 1·5, so that the total mean tumour cell dose would be equivalent to about 4,500 rads of γ-radiation delivered continuously in about 14 days. The minimum tumour cell dose is likely to have a considerably lower value, but it is not possible to estimate this realistically at the present time.

It must be mentioned here that the effective half-life of the tritium of the radioactive drugs in human tumours has a range of values usually between 3 and 14 days. For the bone marrow, whose tritium uptake is low, there is a biphasic biological decrease with values of the half-life of approximately 4 and 13 days. For the kidneys and the small intestine, the half-life is about 8 days. Accordingly, the total radiation dose after intravenous administration of a single dose of 10 curies of e.g. TRK 219 per 70 kg body weight was estimated for the bone marrow 86 $\pm$ 67 rad, and for the kidneys 230 $\pm$ 80 rad (Chipperfield, 1967a). From experience it has been found that an intravenous dose of about 11 curies per 70 kg body weight is without deleterious effects with the proviso that the bone marrow has not been damaged previously, as e.g. by intensive chemotherapy. There is no evidence so far of late damage to the kidneys.

At present instead of large single doses the treatment of choice is the fractionated dosage with repeated intravenous injections of TRK 219 using individual doses of about 3 Ci at time intervals of 3, 4 or 7 days, i.e. usually twice weekly but sometimes once weekly, but often starting with an injection of 1·5 Ci. Usually the total dose administered in the course of intravenous injections amounts to about 20 to 40 Ci per 70 kg body weight.

During this investigation, the use of intra-arterial routes of administration of the radioactive drugs has tended to decrease. It has been useful in selected cases, especially of metastases of melanoma limited to the leg. The method has serious limitations; its success depends both on a high uptake of the radioactive drug into the tumour in the individual patient and on a satisfactory blood supply to the metastases. For example, in a case, Mrs A. M., of recurrent melanoma with multiple metastases involving the left leg, the specific activity of a biopsy specimen from a small metastasis 30 minutes after intra-arterial injection of 7·4 Ci of TRK 219 had the high value of 2·65 mCi per g. Autoradiographs showed a high degree of selective concentration in the tumour with little radioactivity in the stroma; the initial mean dose rate delivered by the tritium in this biopsy specimen was obviously not less than 776 rad per 24 hours. For an assumed value of the biological half-life of 5 days, which is not likely to be an over-estimate, for the corresponding mean life of 7·2 days, the total mean tumour cell dose would be equivalent to not less than about 8,400 rads of γ-radiation delivered continuously in about 7 days. This is a dose within the range of radical treatment. It is interesting to note that many of the small metastases disappeared after the intra-arterial injection but the larger metastases showed at the most only temporary retrogression. The arteriograms showed good vascularity of a small metastasis but deficient blood supply in the large metastasis. It is clear that in this case, the melanoma had a potentially high uptake of the radioactive drug and a sufficiently high level of radiation dose was reached in the small metastases to produce, at least, clinical disappearance of the tumour. However, taking into account the experience of treating several other similar cases of melanoma, it is still an open question whether even after repeated intra-arterial injections, a genuinely curative minimum tumour cell dose has been attained in the smaller metastases. Note must be taken of the probable role of immunity mechanisms in the process of healing in melanoma, after radiotherapy or chemotherapy or very rarely spontaneously. After treatment with TRK 219, there is sometimes a local reaction, which appears to be inflammatory, in and around some of the secondary nodules of melanoma in the skin. This point is made to emphasize the complexity of the therapeutic response to the radioactive drugs, and the limitations of the purely physical approach.

The question must be raised from a general point of view, whether a lethal dose of radiation can be delivered to single tumour cell metastases by any form of administration of these radioactive drugs. Despite the evidence that *in vivo* the uptake of single malignant cells is less than that of the cells in large groups, the possibility of lethal effects on single tumour cells *in vivo* is certainly not excluded, because, in certain cases of advanced malignant tumours of various types, 'tumour-like' cells can be found in the bone marrow, both as isolated cells and in small groups, which concentrate the radioactive drugs (Mitchell, 1966, 1968). It must be added that the identification of these cells is difficult and so far I have not succeeded in studying them by means of electronmicroscopic autoradiography.

It must be recognised that to a large extent, the practical dosage of the radioactive drug has so far been empirical and that much further investigation of dose and time factors is essential, together with studies of methods of increasing the selective uptake into malignant cells. As far as data are available, the clinical results appear to be in general, in agreement with the estimated values of the mean tumour cell dose, on the basis of experience with ordinary radiotherapy. With almost all the patients so far investigated, it has only been possible to give palliative treatments. It is interesting to note that the two cases with long survivals were examples of the radiosensitive neoplastic conditions, testicular seminoma and Hodgkin's disease.

EVIDENCE FROM AUTORADIOGRAPHY

The selective localisation of the tritiated derivatives of MNDP in malignant cells, in contradistinction to the absence of concentration in most normal cells, has been demonstrated directly in many examples of human tumours by means of autoradiography. Details of the technical methods used and a considerable number of examples of the autoradiographs with light microscopy have been published (Mitchell *et al.*, 1963; Mitchell, 1964, 1965a, b, c,

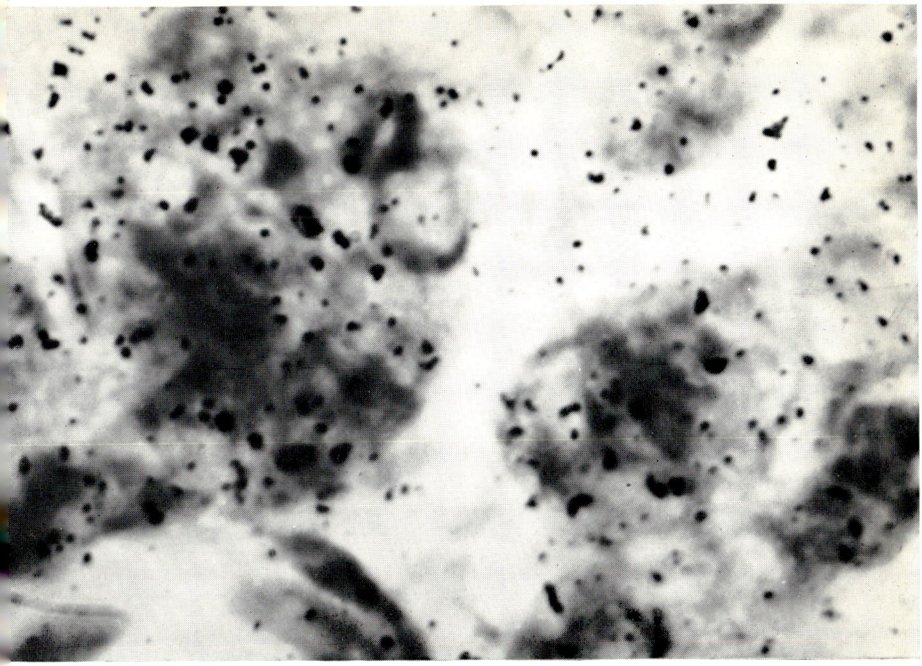

a

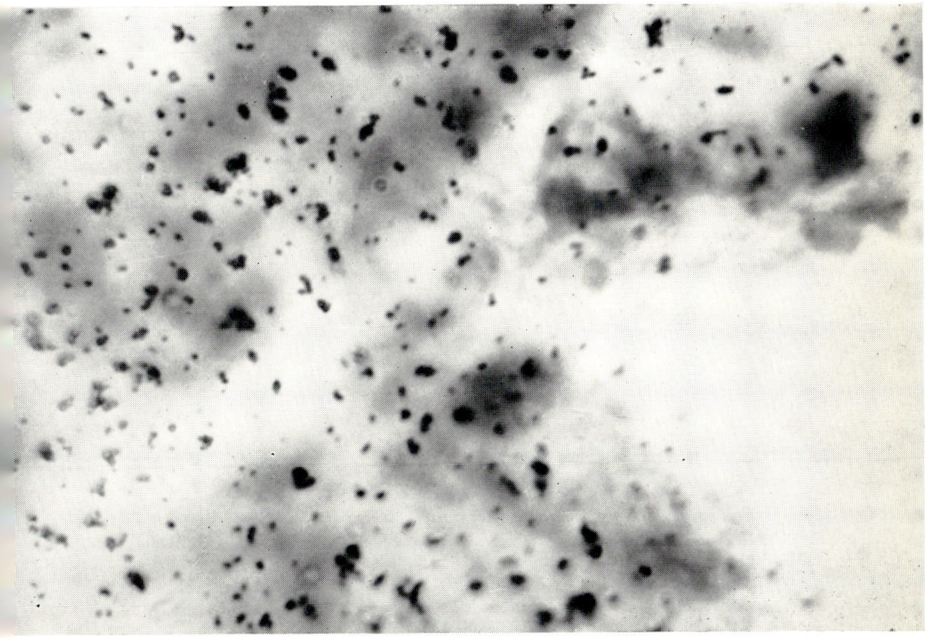

b

ig. 5 Autoradiographs in a case of recurrent melanoma 30 minutes after intravenous injection
4·7 Ci TRK 219. The sections were prepared using freeze-dehydration. Ilford Liquid G5
nulsion. Magnification × 2200. Staining with haematoxylin. Focusing on the silver grains.
(*a*) and (*b*) Subcutaneous metastasis. Exposure time 6 days.

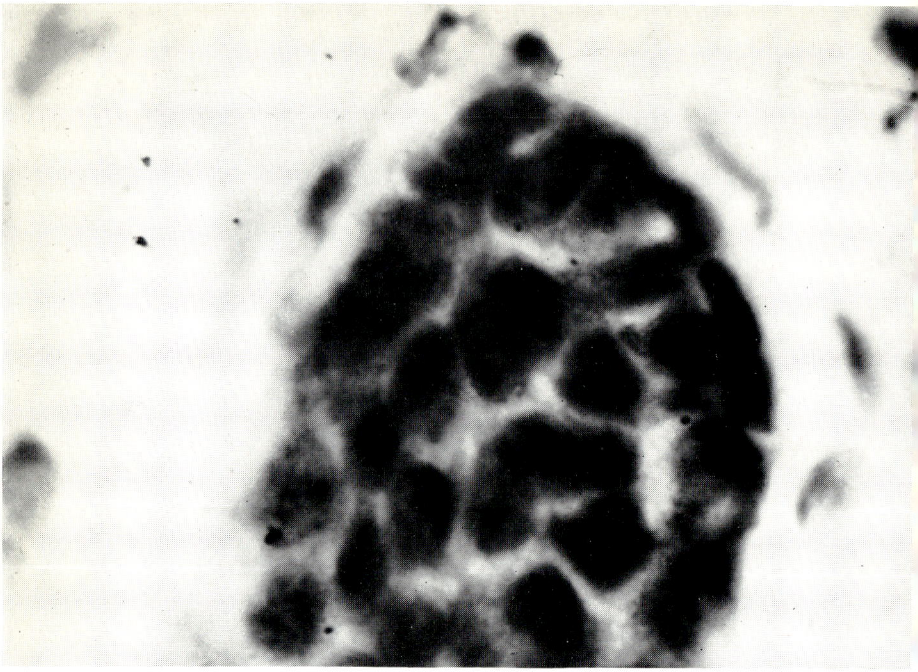

(*c*) Adjacent normal skin. Exposure time 6 days.

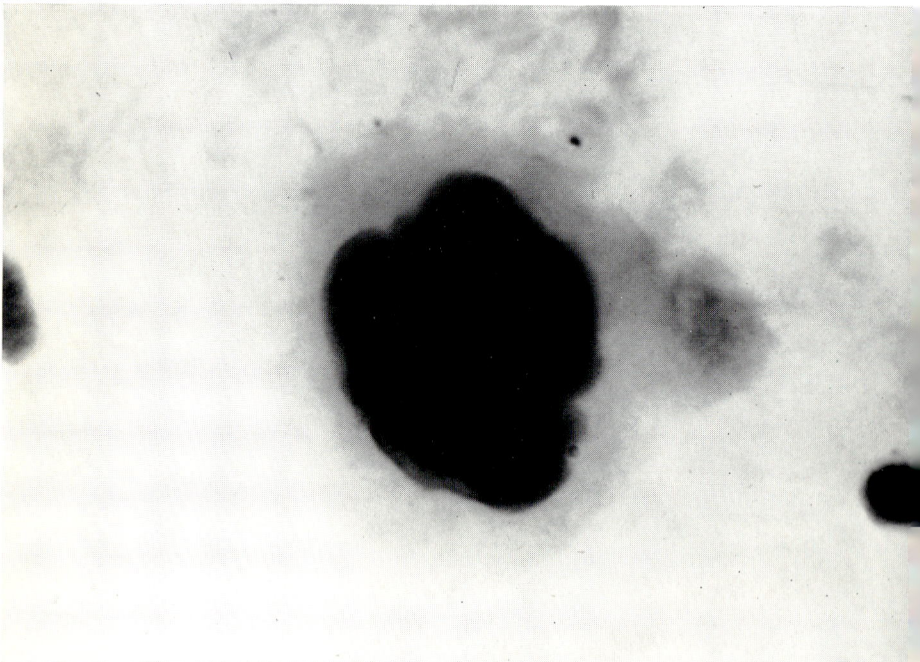

(*d*) Sternal marrow smear, showing megakaryocyte. Exposure time 8 days.

Fig. 5 *continued*

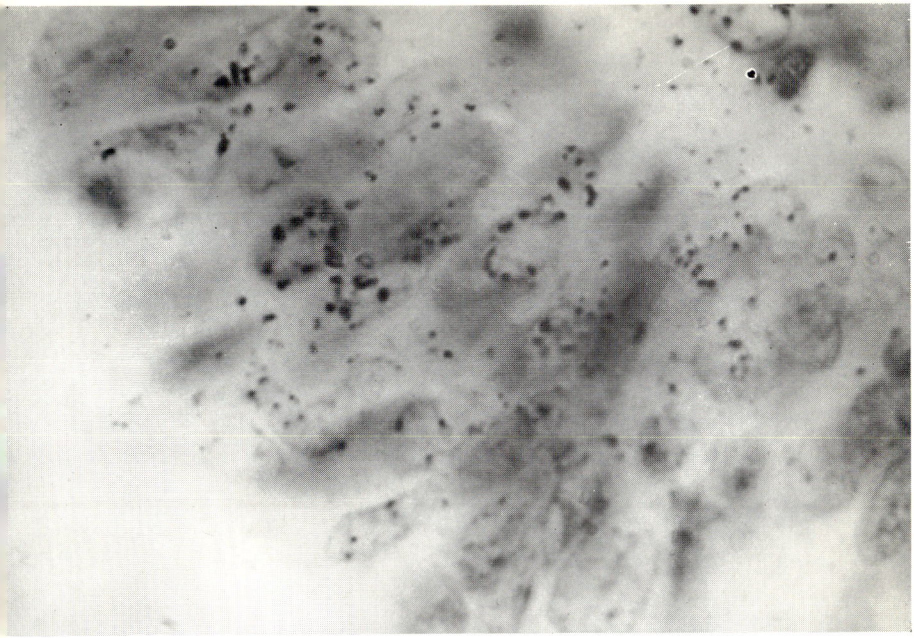

a

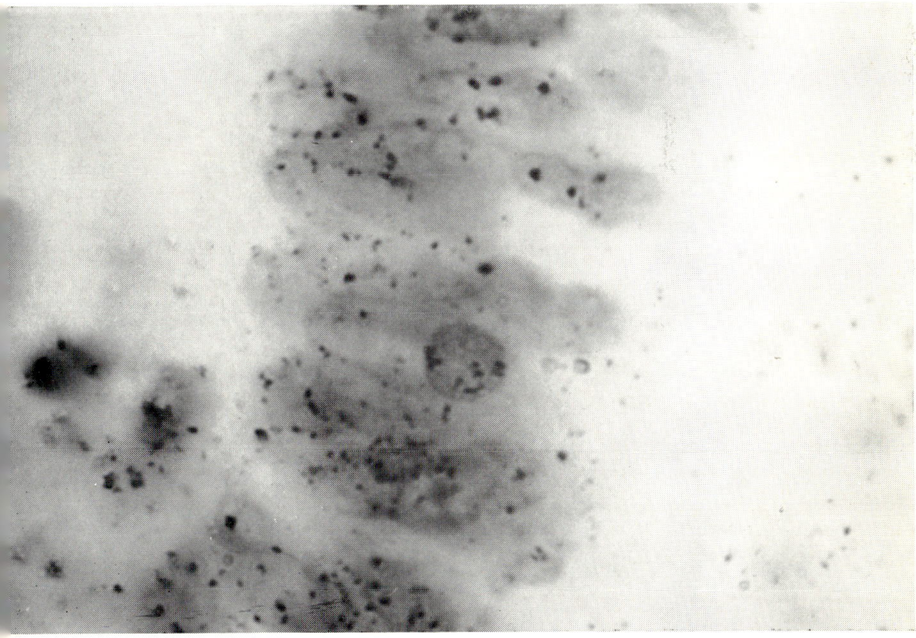

b

g. 6 Autoradiographs of sections of operation specimen of carcinoma of colon, showing the stribution of tritium at 2 hours after intravenous injection of 0·75 Ci TRK 219. Susa fixation, aining with haematoxylin, Ilford G5 liquid emulsion. 7 day autoradiographs. Magnification × 2050. ɔcusing on silver grains.

(*a*) and (*b*) Carcinoma of colon.

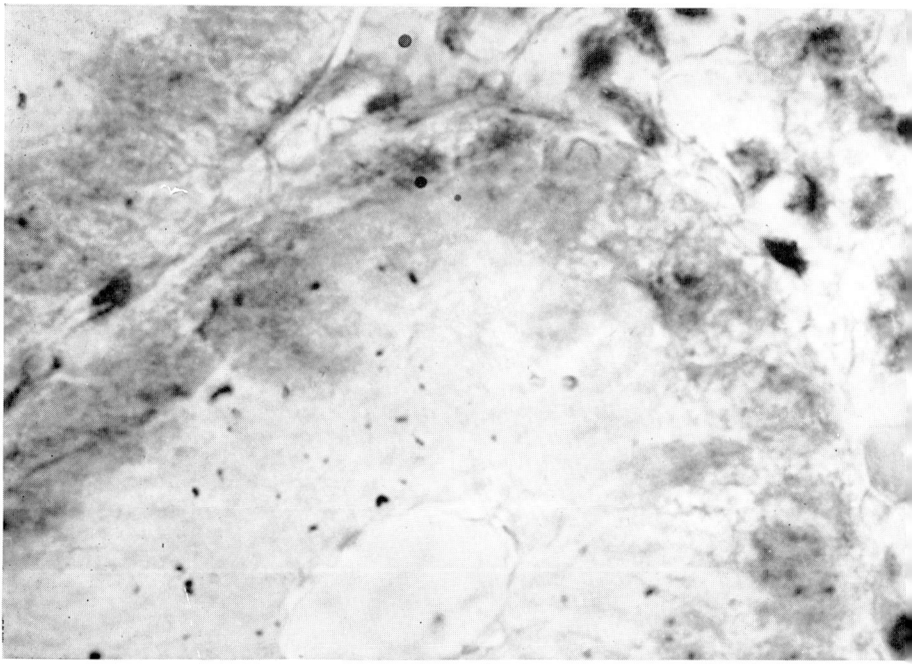

c

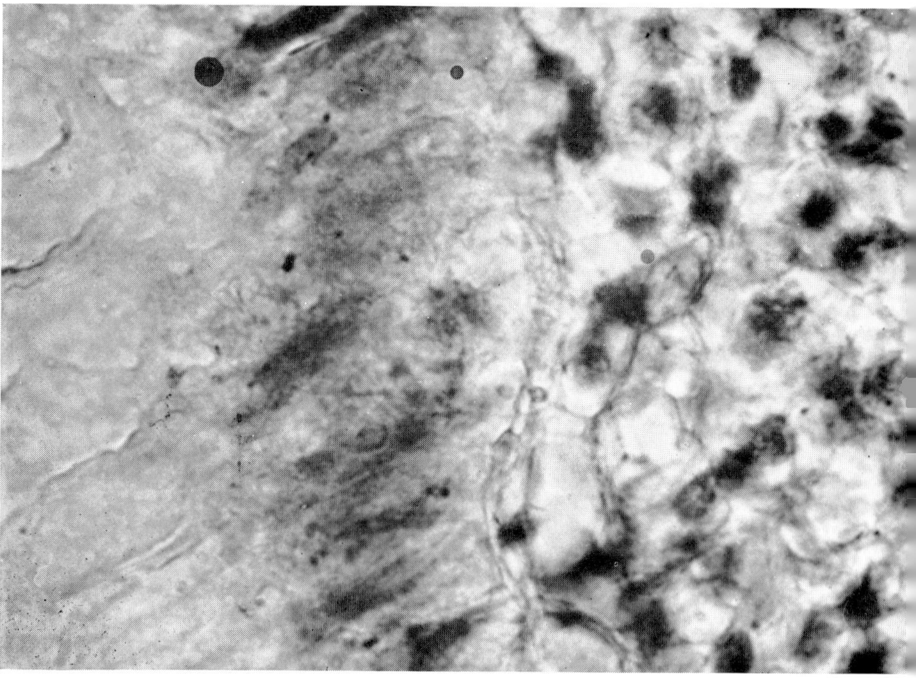

d

Fig. 6 *continued*. (*c*) and (*d*) Adjacent normal colon.

1966, 1967, 1970). For most of this work, the autoradiographs of the histological sections or bone marrow smears were prepared using Ilford G5 fluid emulsion. 5 μ sections were cut after either freeze-drying of Susa fixation of the specimens and embedding in paraffin. The bone marrow smears were dried in air and fixed in methyl alcohol. The optimal exposure times usually varied between 3 and 8 days at 3° C according to the experimental conditions. It is considered that autoradiographic artefact (see e.g. Harbers, 1961) has been excluded by control experiments.

These studies show clearly that the tritium of these radioactive drugs, e.g. TRK 219, is present in the region of the plasma membrane of the cell surface, in the cytoplasm and in the nucleus, particularly in the nucleoli of the tumour cell. With the help of electron microscopic autoradiography it has been found that for tumour cells, the tritium is often outside the cell surface as well as in the immediate region of the plasma membrane, in the cytoplasm, often in the endoplasmic reticulum and sometimes in mitochondria, in the nuclear membrane and finally in the nucleus, particularly in nucleoli, and in relation to nucleolus-associated chromatin and in some areas of heterochromatin. It is of interest that there is practically no labelling of normal lymphocytes. This effect could well be important for the preservation of immunological responses.

We can now consider two examples of typical light microscopic autoradiographs.

(i) The autoradiographs in Fig. 5 were from a biopsy specimen and a sternal marrow smear in a case of recurrent malignant melanoma taken 30 minutes after intravenous injection of 4·7 Ci TRK 219. The tumour cells in the subcutaneous metastasis show a striking concentration of the tritium while the normal cells of the adjacent skin and of the bone marrow show almost no labelling.

(ii) The autoradiographs in Fig. 6, from an operation specimen taken 2 hours after intravenous injection of 0·75 Ci TRK 219, show striking uptake into the adenocarcinoma of the colon but little labelling in any of the cells of the adjacent colon, including lymphocytes.

SOME CONSIDERATIONS OF THE MECHANISMS OF THE THERAPEUTIC ACTIONS OF IONIZING RADIATIONS

Over the years, one of my main aims in research has been to see how far it is possible to understand, and explain quantitatively, the most important mechanisms of the therapeutic actions of ionizing radiations on a molecular and physico-chemical basis.

The difficulties of the subject are due to the extraordinary complexity of biological processes. In this field consideration must be given to biological variability, homeostatic mechanisms – to maintain the constancy of the internal environment – changes in response to injury, including host responses, and, last but not least, repair and reconstructive processes at all levels of organisation. Some of the most important problems involve the differences in the radiosensitivity of different types of living cells for a particular defined biological effect.

Specifically, our immediate concern is to study the mechanisms by which measured doses of ionizing radiations, mainly X- and γ- and β-rays, act upon the cells of a malignant tumour and the adjacent and interwoven normal cells and tissues, and upon the patient as a whole. Of practical relevance is the need to understand both the differences between the malignant cells of human tumours and the normal cells of the body as the basis for the curability of certain tumours by radiotherapy and the nature of the differences between radiocurable and radio-incurable tumours. Quantitative studies of mammalian cells *in vitro* have proved to be important. However, a great deal of relevant quantitative evidence has been obtained by the study of simpler organisms, especially bacteria. The limitations of biological knowledge must be emphasised, despite the remarkable advances in molecular biology. In fact, a valuable use of radiations has been its application as a tool for the investigation of cells. I always hope that knowledge of the mechanisms of the therapeutic actions of ionizing radiations will contribute toward the provision of a rational basis for the development of the chemotherapy of neoplastic diseases.

I have considered this subject in a number of reviews (Mitchell, 1966, 1968a and b) and will concentrate here on the problem of the role of deoxyribonucleic acid, DNA. (See also Hutchinson, 1966.) As I have already mentioned, it seems that there is substantial evidence in support of the conclusion that a 'macromolecular lesion' of DNA in the nucleoprotein system of the living cell, with unrepaired damage, is the basis for the injury to malignant cells by radiation, which leads to their death as a result of radiotherapy (Mitchell, 1955, 1956, 1960, 1966). Further, I have suggested that the macromolecular lesion of DNA, relevant in radiotherapy, is a break involving both strands of the double helical structure, which is not repaired (Mitchell, 1968a, b, c). Reference may be made here to the review by Swingle and Cole (1968) in which the following conclusion is reached. 'The changes occurring in lymphocytes and other mammalian cells which die in interphase after relatively low doses of ionizing radiation are probably initiated by the same types of damage to DNA as that which results in reproductive death of proliferating cells'.

It must be pointed out that this mechanism is by no means generally accepted. There is extensive evidence that radiosensitisation of cells is produced by the thymidine analogues, 5-bromo- and 5-iodo-deoxyuridine, after incorporation into the DNA. (See review by Kaplan, 1970.) At least superficially, these findings provide strong support for the conclusion that DNA is the principal target in the killing of mammalian cells by X- and

γ- and β-rays. Nevertheless, it appears that incorporation of the halogenated base analogues impairs or suppresses the post-irradiation repair of DNA (Lett, Parkins, Alexander and Ormerod, 1964; Aoki, Boyce and Howard-Flanders, 1966; Fox and Lajtha, 1967; Fox, 1968; Lett, Caldwell and Little, 1970). The problem is complex and difficult, particularly because as yet, there is much less evidence concerning strand breakage, degradation and repair of DNA in mammalian cells than in bacteria. In the important experiments of McGrath *et coll.* (McGrath, Williams and Swartz-endruber, 1966; McGrath and Williams, 1966) with exponentially growing cells of two strains of Escherichia coli, B/r, the strain resistant to radiation had D_{37} about 15 kR and the radiosensitive strain, B_{s-1}, a value of D_{37} about 3 kR. The molecular weight of the DNA obtained from both strains was reduced to the same extent by a dose of 20 kR. However, after 40 minutes incubation at 38° C, the molecular weight of the DNA from the irradiated radioresistant bacteria had returned to nearly the normal value while that from the radiosensitive organisms had not. Of even greater importance is the repair of X-ray damage to DNA demonstrated by Lett, Feldschreiber, Little, Steele and Dean, 1967 (see also Moseley and Laser, 1965) in the extraordinarily radioresistant bacterium *Micrococcus radiodurans*, which under anoxic conditions completely survives doses of up to 500 krads. The DNA of this organism has much the same radiosensitivity as that of mouse lymphoma cells (Lett *et al.*, 1967; Alexander *et al.*, 1970) but in *M. radiodurans* repair processes are extremely efficient and in addition it appears that the cells contain a natural radioprotecting substance (Bruce and Malchman, 1965). Measurements of the inactivation doses for *E. coli* exposed to α-particles, protons of different LETs and γ-rays have been interpreted by target theory in terms of two types of lethal damage to the genome (Munson *et al.*, 1967); these workers consider that 'it is quite probable that type 1 and type 2 lesions are identical with those which can be observed *in vitro* as single- and double-strand breaks. However, simple application of oxygen enhancement values for single and double-strand breaks in free DNA leads to a prediction contrary to observation (Alper, 1968; Munson *et al.*, 1968). Recently evidence has been presented concerning modification by chemical agents of post-irradiation degradation of DNA in *E. coli* B/r, which leads to the conclusion that 'there are strong indications that DNA is not the only or even the most important target for the killing of bacteria by ionizing radiation'. (Cramp, 1970; see also Alper, 1961, 1963, 1968; Pollard and Weller, 1968.)

In bacteriophages, there is some precise information but there are still problems. The yield of breaks in the DNA after irradiation can be measured more accurately in phages than in bacteria, because the molecules are smaller and less susceptible to damage during extraction, and further the DNA can be separated more easily from the protein. One cannot completely exclude the possibility that the isolation procedure leads to the breaking of bonds which have been labelled by the action of radiation. It has been shown by Freifelder (1968) that 'when phages λ, T5 and T7 are inactivated by X-irradiation, approximately half the lethal events are double-strand breaks and half are presumably some type of base damage. However, in the phage T4 almost all of the lethal events are double strand-breaks'. Recently for DNA-isolated after irradiation of T4 or T7 bacteriophage with γ-rays – and analysed for double and single-strand breaks by sedimentation in a sucrose gradient – van der Schans and Blok (1970) found that in the absence of oxygen, the number of double-strand breaks per krad and per molecular weight of 10^9 daltons is 0·04, and in the presence of oxygen is 0·08. The yield of single strand breaks is 10 to 20 times higher than that of double-strand breaks. (See also Weinert and Hagen, 1968.) It was shown that the increase in DNA breaks in the presence of oxygen does not manifest itself as an increased sensitivity of the bacteriophage as a whole, because the presence of oxygen prevents other types of damage, presumably in the protein coat. If sulphydryl compounds are present, the yield of DNA breaks is not much affected, but the amount of other damage is considerably reduced and a normal oxygen effect is observed.

In general terms, it appears to be a useful concept that therapeutic doses of ionizing radiations produce lesions of certain macromolecular systems *in vivo* and *in vitro.* It must be emphasised that this is not the whole story and only part of the explanation of the biochemical effects of ionizing radiations, see e.g. my review (Mitchell, 1966) and the books by Bacq and Alexander (1961) and Streffer (1969).

Lesions of extra-cellular macromolecules in the matrix of connective tissues are of considerable interest in radiobiology and can be attributed to depolymerisation and degradation of glycosaminoglycans (mucopolysaccharides), especially hyaluronic acid. These processes are often extremely radiosensitive both *in vivo* in the dermis and in connective tissues generally and *in vitro* and can be observed after doses as small as 20–50 rads (Brinkman and Lamberts, 1968; 1960; 1966). They are anomalous, from the point of view of radiobiology, in that oxygen has either no influence on them or confers protection against radiation, instead of sensitising. Experiments using the methods of pulse radiolysis have shown that the sensitivity of hyaluronic acid in aqueous solution to radiation damage is due to 'facile reactions with both major products of water radiolysis e_{aq-} and OH' (Balazs, Davies, Phillips and Young, 1967).

Returning to the complex problem of the role of DNA in the mechanisms of the therapeutic actions of X and γ-radiations on human tumour cells, it is perhaps simplest to consider the evidence historically. At therapeutic levels of dosage, a disturbance of cellular nucleic acid metabolism with accumulation of pentose nucleotides and RNA and inhibition of synthesis of DNA was demonstrated (Mitchell, 1940, 1942a, b, c, 1943, 1944) mainly in human tumours but also in the Jensen rat sarcoma, by the use of ultra-violet photomicrography combined with photographic photometry and histochemical studies. As is well known, Euler and Hevesy (1942, 1944) using ^{32}P labelled phosphate as a tracer demonstrated a reduction in the formation of DNA in the Jensen rat sarcoma after X-irradiation with doses of 1,000 R and less of X-rays. Other studies on tumour cells using ultraviolet microspectroscopy were reported by Caspersson, Klein and Ringertz (1958) and Killander, Richards and Ringertz (1962). The cytoplasmic accumulation of RNA after irradiation was confirmed and studied intensively by Seed (1966), who found that about half the accumulation of cytoplasmic RNA was inhibited when DNA synthesis was blocked. It is of interest that recently Hidvegi *et al.* (1970) demonstrated an increase in DNA-dependent RNA synthesis in the guinea-pig liver after whole body irradiation with a dose of 2,000 rads of X-rays. Treatment of the animals with actinomycin D shortly before irradiation abolished the radiation-induced enrichment of polysomes and the increase in protein synthesis.

Following up my own early work, I calculated using simple assumptions that in the treatment of a small human squamous carcinoma of the skin with a single dose of 2,000 R of X-rays, one ion pair stops the formation of one molecule of DNA of molecular weight about 6×10^6 (Mitchell, 1955). 'The possibility of a direct action mechanism in DNA or DNA-protein must be raised. It may be suggested that damage anywhere in the DNA molecule stops self-duplication'. Later it was suggested that the killing of tumour cells in radiotherapy was based on the production of a 'macromolecular lesion' involving DNA in the deoxyribonucleoprotein system of the nucleus (Mitchell, 1956; see also 1960). For some years it was generally considered that no changes could be detected in the physical properties of DNA isolated from mammalian cells *in vivo*. However, Harbers and Backmann (1956) demonstrated a large increase in the fraction of DNA of lower molecular weight in the Walker rat carcinosarcoma two hours after irradiation with a dose of 5,000 R of X-rays. Of great interest is the work of Strazhevskaya and Struchkov (1962, 1963) who used extremely gentle techniques for the isolation of DNA from tissues and obtained preparations of such high viscosity that they did not commit themselves as to whether these contained single molecules or complexes, but termed them 'supramolecular'. 'It is shown that immediately after γ-irradiation of rats we can observe a well-defined disruption of the state of the supramolecular structures in thymus and liver'. In the preparations from normal liver, recovery of the viscosity occurred, e.g. at 6 hours after a dose of 1000 R.

Of great radiobiological interest is the effect of relatively small doses of X-radiation *in vivo* on the nucleoproteins of the highly radiosensitive cells of the mammalian thymus gland. Hagen (1960) demonstrated 'labilisation' of DNA in thymus nucleoprotein after whole-body irradiation of rats, even with doses of 50 R and 100 R. Increased extractability of DNA is observed at times of more than 1 hour after irradiation *in vivo*. The maximum yield of DNA is about 50% and is obtained at about 6 hours after irradiation with doses of 400–800 R of X-radiation using 1% trichloracetic acid in the phenol-trichloracetic acid extraction procedure. It is to be noted that the DNA and proteins separated after irradiation can be re-associated by the addition of calcium ions or magnesium ions (Hagen, 1960). A close similarity was found between the decrease of specific viscosity of the DNA extracted from the thymus at different times after irradiation *in vivo* and the proportion of cells with pyknotic and presumably irreversibly damaged nuclei (Hagen, 1961).

Reference must be made to the related study by Ernst (1961) of the early loss of the proteins of the thymus cell nucleus after total body irradiation with a dose of 1000 R. The first change after irradiation is loss of about half of the globulin fraction of the nucleus in the first half-hour; loss of the histone fraction occurs more slowly and to a lesser extent. These changes reach their maximum at about 1 hour after 1,000 R, when the extractability of the DNA starts to increase.

In the comparison of the decrease of nucleoprotein in the cell nuclei of thymus, spleen and liver (Ernst, 1963), loss of nucleoprotein occurred during the first 4 hours in the nuclei of all three tissues, but later gradual recovery occurred in the radioresistant liver cell nuclei.

In recent studies of DNA-histone interactions in deoxyribonucleoprotein isolated from the rat thymus after total body irradiation with 1,000 R of X-rays Bauer, Johansen, and Thomasson (1969), concluded that 'alterations in the histones appear to be correlated with degradation of the DNA'. The next step is to consider to radiosensitivity of mammalian cells quantitatively. There is, of course, a great deal of evidence available (see Hewitt, 1963; Whitmore and Till, 1964) concerning the effects of radiation in producing loss of the capacity of single cells to proliferate – or loss of reproductive integrity, as it was termed by Gray (1959) – following the elegant methods of the study of clone cultures introduced by Puck, Marcus and Cieciura (1956). Although there is a considerable spread in the observed values of the parameters of the dose-effect curves, it is a reasonably good approximation for many mammalian cells that at least when well oxygenated, the value of D_{37} – the dose for 37% (1/e) survival suitably defined – is about 140 rads, while under anoxic conditions D_{37} often has a value of about 350 rads; the observed value of the intercept at zero dose, now generally termed the extrapolation number, is often close to 2. There is, however, evidence that under strictly anoxic conditions, the extrapolation number is approximately unity (Révész and Littbrand, 1966, 1967). The biological picture is complicated further by the influence of irradiation on growth rate and clone size (see Nias, Gilbert, Lajtha and Lange, 1965) and the survival of cells, e.g. HeLa cells, after large doses of radiation (Lund and Rosengren, 1966). Moreover, treatment of the dose-effect curves by means of the theory of Atwood and Norman (1949) has inevitable limitations and it is necessary to consider the problem in much greater detail. In their book, Hug and Kellerer (1966) introduce the concept of relative steepness, of the dose-effect curve, defined by $S = \overline{D}^2/\sigma^2$, where $\overline{D}$ is the *mean* inactivation dose and σ^2 its variance. Proof is given of the theorem that if a dose-effect relation has the relative steepness S, the mean number, ν, of absorption events which are necessary to produce the observed effect is at least S. For example, the data of Humphrey and Sinclair (1963) for the Lettré-Ehrlich ascites tumour cells *in vitro* gave a value of D_{37} of 405 rads with extrapolation number 6, but the value of S was found to be 3·9 with $\bar{D} = 379$ rads; in this case, at least four independent elementary processes are necessary for the death of the cells.

The uncertainties are so great that only order of magnitude calculations are of immediate interest. At the risk of over-simplification and omission of the discussion of factors thought not to be of immediate relevance, it is useful to examine the results of an elementary presentation of the application of target theory to this problem (see Mitchell, 1960, p. 26; 1966, p. 448; 1968). For a target of molecular weight M daltons and D_{37} in rad, and taking into account the energy yield, G, which is the number of molecules changed per 100 eV absorbed, it is found that

$$MD_{37} = 0{\cdot}965 \times 10^{12}/G$$

It may be assumed for a typical tumour cell in the presence of oxygen that the value of D_{37} is 140 rad. Accordingly, the lethal action behaves as if it results from damage to macromolecular units of molecular weight in the region of $0{\cdot}7 \times 10^{10}$ daltons for $G = 1$ and $0{\cdot}7 \times 10^{11}$ for $G = 1/10$.

Under anoxic conditions, it may be assumed that the value of D_{37} is 350 rad. If it is assumed, as will be discussed below, that in fact the target is to be identified with DNA and that the relevant macromolecular lesion is a unrepaired double break, it is possible to assume a G value of 0·031 as determined by Weinert and Hagen (1968) for moist calf-thymus deoxyribonucleoprotein gel of concentration 20% irradiated in nitrogen with γ-rays. The corresponding value of the target weight would be $0{\cdot}9 \times 10^{11}$. It must be assumed that for each cell, inactivation of a small number, perhaps 2 or 4, independent targets is necessary for the lethal effect.

For some years, it has been reasonably certain that the DNA of the nuclei of mammalian cells is of very high molecular weight and great chain length and the possibility has often been discussed that a single DNA molecule extends throughout the whole length of a chromosome, obviously with some compact form of coiling and probably with multiple spiralisation (see Lampert, 1969).

If this picture is correct, the molecular weight of the DNA would be in the region of 10^{10} to 10^{11} daltons; if there were 2, 4 or 8 molecules per chromosome the value of the molecular weight would be reduced accordingly. It is possible that the radiosensitive structure is some type of coiled chain of long sub-units of macromolecular DNA, joined together by very short and possibly fragile links, perhaps of non-histone protein – and functioning in the cell as an essential biological unit. In the classical autoradiographic studies of the DNA of HeLa cells, Cairns (1966) showed that at least 100 units of DNA that are duplicated individually and simultaneously appear to be joined in series to form a much longer structure. It is simplest to conclude that the critical radiosensitive structure is a single continuous macromolecule of DNA weight in the region of 10^{10} to 10^{11} daltons. These are truly giant macromolecules; it is interesting to mention that DNA of molecular weight $1{\cdot}9_2 \times 10^{10}$ has a chain length of 1 cm. It appeared to be reasonable to assume that the relevant radiation lesion of the DNA is a break involving both strands of the double helical structure which is not repaired, and the experimental evidence now available appears to support this conclusion. The break in the DNA structure must occur at random throughout the whole molecule, even though at one of a large number of similar vulnerable sites, and must inactivate the molecule as a whole. The assumption of a ring structure for the DNA would give a simple explanation for the inactivation of the whole molecule by a single random lesion. In the mammalian cell covalently circular DNA is possible, but completion of the ring by some other molecular structure should also be considered. These considerations involve many difficult theoretical problems, including the role of the nucleolus – which has been shown to be more radiosensitive than the rest of the nucleus in elegant X-ray microbeam irradiation experiments by Seed (1960). Detailed investigation will be necessary to study the apparent lack of significant effects of single strand breaks and base damage, and of cross-linking.

Experimental evidence in support of the main conclusions has appeared in recent years. Lett and Alexander (1966) reported as follows: 'After lymphoma cells have been given a dose of 5,000 R, their DNA is reduced to a molecular weight of 3×10^8 (single stranded) and this can be readily measured. With increasing doses of radiation, the molecular weight falls further and the reciprocal of the molceular weight is proportional to the radiation dose . . .'. After 1,000 R the molecular weight corresponds to 2×10^9 (double stranded) (Alexander, 1967; see also Lett, Caldwell, Dean and Alexander, 1967). Extrapolation to zero dose indicates that the molecular weight of the DNA in the unirradiated lymphoma cell is greater than 10^{10}. It is interesting to note that the curves for irradiation under oxygen and nitrogen extrapolate at zero dose to give the same value of the weight-average molecular weight of the DNA.

Until recently, direct measurement of the molecular weight of the target DNA of mammalian cells did not seem possible. (For some time I have been trying to study this problem by means of autoradiography with thymidine labelling of the DNA of Ehrlich ascites tumour cells and also electron microscopy using sedimentation under gravity – as a poor man's method.)

An experiment which appears to be decisive, has been carried out in Japan by Terasima and Tsuboi (1969). Long pieces of DNA were isolated from cultured mouse L5 cells by sedimentation. The cultures had been fed with tritiated thymidine to label the DNA. The isolation procedure consisted of a simple deproteinisation of the cells and handling with minimal shearing. The sedimentation constant ($S_{20,w}$) of the DNA isolated from unirradiated cells was estimated to be approximately 330S; the corresponding value of the molecular weight, calculated with certain assumptions was about 2×10^{10}. The sedimentation profile of the tritium was demonstrated consistently. The sedimentation behaviour of the DNA molecules obtained from irradiated cells provided a sensitive measure for detecting double strand breaks. The strands were isolated soon after irradiation of the cells with 200 kV X-rays of HVL 1·2 mmCu at a dose of 490 rads per minute. The doses used included 2·8, 7·5 and 9·4 krads. As the dose increased, a shift of the profile toward the meniscus was demonstrated. The ratio of sedimentation distance of the DNA from irradiated cells to that of the unirradiated control when plotted against X-ray dose, showed a simple exponential decrease starting from the origin, with a few points well below the line. Quoting from this paper: 'Assuming the molecular weight of 2×10^{10} daltons for the DNA of L5 cells, a nucleus of the cell should contain about 450 molecules. Since each molecule will have one break, on the average, after an exposure of 7·5 krads, about 17 rads would be necessary to cause one break per nucleus. Thus, it may be that about 10 breaks of the double-stranded DNA are needed for the death of L5 cells whose mean lethal dose, D_0, was determined to be approximately 175 rads. If the estimate of molecular weight is larger than the real value, more breaks would be responsible for the mitotic death of L5 cells'.

Further work is needed in this field and it is my view that its study is likely to be of considerable value, both scientifically and practically. It is obviously necessary to find out whether there is any correlation between the radiosensitivity of cells, both normal and malignant, and the molecular weight of the relevant DNA. The existence of a linear relationship between the molecular weight and $1/D_{37}$ is not impossible, but it is clear that many other factors play an important role, including oxygen tension, sulphydryl groups and chromosome structure and complement. In recent years it has come to be recognised that large differences in apparent radiosensitivity are introduced by recovery and reconstructive processes after irradiation. The whole of this subject is complicated and it is by no means impossible that the processes are different in bacteria and in mammalian cells.

The question of possible differences in the structure of DNA between normal and malignant cells is obviously important and immediately relevant to the problems of radiosensitivity and radiocurability. It is my own view that logical consideration of the scientific evidence from many fields leads to the conclusion that alterations in the structure of DNA are the most likely basis for malignancy. This hypothesis should be either proved or disproved by further experimental studies, probably with the aid of new techniques. It may be of interest to mention that recently, Webb and Bather (1970) found evidence from infra-red spectra of normal and tumour DNA at different levels of relative humidity, suggesting that the conformation of the tumour DNA 'seems to be fixed permanently between the B and A forms'. Further, DNA isolated from a premalignant lesion of the liver induced in rats by the carcinogen, 2-fluorenylacetamide, was found by Epstein *et al.* (1970) to show obvious alterations in its chemical and physical properties, including 'denatured and distorted fibres as observed with electron microscopy, when compared with DNA from normal control liver, the surrounding non-hyperplastic liver or regenerating liver following partial hepatectomy'. This is an exciting field at the present time.

IV

If curable, why not cured?

A PARTIAL ANSWER TO THE QUESTION AND SOME PROBLEMS OF ORGANISATION

To put the question in perspective, we must come back to the patient. I think it is useful to consider the problem of patients with cancer and the study of malignant diseases, a subject which is now sometimes given the name 'oncology', as an example of a major branch of medicine and medical science in the wide sense.

We have seen that at present, in this country, of all the patients treated with cancer and allied diseases – excluding 'rodent ulcer', which is curable – it is reasonable to estimate that about one-quarter are cured in the sense of surviving with a normal expectation of life. The main methods of treatment, surgery, radiotherapy, and chemotherapy and combinations of these, with immunotherapy emerging, are not rivals but must all be used as necessary to the best advantage of the individual patient. When cure is not possible, the tremendous value of palliative treatment in relieving unpleasant symptoms, especially pain, and often in restoring the patient to normal health for a time, must be emphasised. After palliative treatment many patients learn to live normal lives again, even for some years; this can be very important particularly if it comes at the time when the patient's young children are growing up. Quoting from the World Health Organisation Technical Report No. 322 (1966): 'It has indeed been estimated that one cancer in every three is of a type for which cure by the best existing methods is feasible. This hopeful aspect of cancer is insufficiently appreciated, even by the medical profession itself; too many pessimistic patients find themselves consulting equally pessimistic physicians'. Lack of confidence in the value of treatment, associated with deeply ingrained fears and anxieties often conspire to prevent prompt action being taken to diagnose and treat people with cancer. To some extent these difficulties are slowly being overcome. A better standard of general education and the popularisation of medical information are making it possible for cancer to be talked about to a greater extent as an ordinary disease. Even more important are the steadily improving methods of diagnosis, treatment and care and the greater psychological understanding of the patient and his or her problems. I would like to suggest that it is vital that not only the patients and of course the doctors, but also the administrators, should realise what can be done. It is perhaps inevitable that many people only appreciate both the good and the bad sides of the problem when they and their own families are involved.

At the present time, the practical utilisation, as far as possible, of the facilities and knowledge available is essential, but the most important factor limiting the improvement of the diagnosis and treatment of patients with cancer and the prevention of cancer is *lack of knowledge*. In my opinion, there is an urgent need for much more clinical and laboratory research in relation to the cancer field, not only what is called in current jargon 'mission oriented' research but also fundamental and 'curiosity based' research.

Medical services, medical research and medical education are linked to the economy as a whole. The problem of cancer must be considered in this context, however much one may deplore what one of my colleagues called 'assessing the value of human life in terms of money'; the occasion was when I mentioned that I understood that the Library of the Ministry of Health has bought a copy of my book '*Studies in Radiotherapeutics*' (1960, see p. 183) primarily for the table of 'Comparison of costs of treatment per patient with different types of apparatus' for radiotherapy. To the doctor, the welfare and happiness of his individual patient must be the first consideration and it is exasperating to him that shortage of money should limit the facilities available. Quite apart from any question of human happiness, prevention of cancer is cheapest, and it now looks as if this will be imporatnt in the case of cancer of the uterine cervix, despite the difficulties of this problem. Of the value of curative treatment, there can be no doubt. It is my considered opinion, that even from the most hard-headed point of view of costs, it is economically advantageous in the long term to give the best possible palliative treatment to patients with cancer, who cannot be cured. In discussing this subject, I wish to emphasise that I have always felt that in this country and despite the shortage of money available the Ministry of Health (now the Department of Health and Social Security) has done its best and in fact accomplished a great deal, with genuine human understanding. None-the-less, I could not have provided the facilities we have available for the treatment of patients with cancer here in Cambridge without substantial help from outside the National Health Service.

In considering the even more complex problem of research in the cancer field, I would like to mention first the difficulties and delay in the practical application of the results of research. Even if a 'breakthrough' were made today and its potential importance recognised immediately, it would probably take at least 10 years to bring it into general use. It is of interest to take note of the report entitled 'An attempt to quantify the economic benefits of scientific research' by Byatt and Cohen (1969). The basic idea is that much pure or 'curiosity-oriented' research pursued for its own sake in or around universities and Research Council laboratories, tends to give rise to major industries in about a generation or less. The nature of such industries could not have been predicted at the time of the basic scientific discovery. The aim of cancer research is essentially different but the problems of the relative values of the practical benefits of applied and fundamental research will, inevitably I think, be considered along similar lines. We have already mentioned the time-lag in the application of radium, discovered in 1898, in the treatment of cancer of the uterine cervix. It took 10 years, from 1903 to 1913, before its value in the curative treatment of technically operable cases was recognised. Only after another 10–15 years were the 5-year results published for a number of large series of cases. In other examples, the application of the cytology of smears to the detection of precancerous lesions of the uterine cervix, the basic scientific work on mice and rabbits was published by Stockhard and Papanicolaou in 1917. In the search for human cancer cells, Papanicolaou (1928) was the first to grasp the significance of exfoliative cytology. The method was launched into clinical practice after the publication in 1943 of the book '*Diagnosis of Uterine Cancer*' by Papanicolaou and Traut.

It is difficult to take account of rare and very important discoveries, such as that of radium, except to realise that such events can occur, and are perhaps most likely to occur, in the course of research in entirely unrelated fields. As far as policy based on prediction is concerned, it is my view that in the United Kingdom both applied and fundamental research in the cancer field and in associated sciences of possible relevance, should be encouraged by the increasing financial support, mainly of interested university departments and also of a number of existing research institutes. For the country as a whole, my own estimate of the best ratio of research regarded as applied to that regarded as fundamental is about 4 to 1, but in giving this figure it must be emphasised that the distinction between the two types is less clear than in the consideration of relevance to industrial developments. Although it may be considered that the cost is too great, I think it is highly desirable that the U.K. should have a National Cancer Institute. It is my view that this should be associated with an established general hospital, with a radiotherapeutic centre serving a large population, and with a University with a medical school. I personally think it is advantageous for most non-medical scientists working in the cancer field to have some contact with the clinical problems of cancer and frequent opportunities to discuss their problems with the clinicians. It is essential to provide substantially greater opportunities for first-class scientists coming from a wide range of disciplines to make an attractive career in the general field of cancer. At the present time, especially with the technological gap between the U.S.A. and the U.K., we must make full use of our knowledge and resources and, moreover, we must provide a much more stimulating climate in which to discover new facts and exploit and develop new ideas.

I think that the interested medical and scientific departments of at least some universities in the U.K. should play a greater part in the study of cancer, given increased financial support. It is now widely accepted that this subject is a proper field for academic study. As an example, I would like to give a brief account of my own approach to these problems. I have built up a close association between the Hospital and the University and between the clinical and laboratory work, particularly from the point of view of research and development. The policy of having both the clinic and at least some of the laboratories close together in the same building has been of great help in achieving this. Over the years, the staff of the Department of Radiotherapeutics and of the Radiotherapeutic Centre at Addenbrooke's Hospital, Cambridge, have worked together as a team.

As a University Clinical Department, the Department of Radiotherapeutics has three main types of activity and responsibility, which must be considered separately, though they are closely inter-related.

(1) First and foremost, the care, diagnosis, investigation and treatment of patient, who in this department are largely, though by no means exclusively, patients with malignant diseases and allied conditions.

(2) Teaching, which in this case is mainly postgraduate and may be summarised as clinical training and research with personal supervision, together with regular clinical staff meetings and seminars and a limited number of formal lectures.

(3) Research and development, the ultimate aim of which is to improve the treatment of patients with cancer. Fundamental research has always been regarded as one of the essential activities of the department and particular attention has been paid to studies of the mechanisms of the therapeutic actions of radiations. Over the door of the laboratories I put up the motto 'The aim of this department is to improve the treatment of cancer'.

It must be emphasised that the care of the individual patient as a whole is the foundation of the work of the department. It has always been made clear that in this department, radiotherapeutics is regarded as a branch of general medicine concerned with the treatment of patients with neoplastic diseases and that all methods of treatment including the chemotherapy of cancer are important in its activities. I have often made the point that a great deal of knowledge in the field of radiotherapy should be integrated into general medicine.

I would now like to say a few words about two topics which I think are important.

(1) *The treatment of the individual patient*

I feel that to do one's duty as a doctor, one must aim at medical treatment, including radiotherapy, and chemotherapy, which is 'patient-oriented' and not 'disease-oriented'. I have done my best to provide individualised treatment, both curative and palliative with total care of the patient and continued advice and support for his family. This approach involves a substantial and sustained effort, but I have no doubt that it is abundantly worth while from the point of view of the patient and in terms of human welfare, even though this is difficult to express statistically.

I think that many doctors, including myself, practise the treatment of patients with cancer, including radiotherapy and chemotherapy, with some understanding of the place of surgery, as a branch of internal medicine. It seems to me that serious consideration should be given to recognition of this field as medical speciality. It might be called 'medical oncology'.

I have come to the conclusion that in this country it is advantageous that a radiotherapeutic centre or a centre for the treatment of patients with cancer should be part of the complex of a large general hospital, which should be a teaching hospital associated with a university. It is interesting that this conclusion was reached many years ago by Forssell (1930 and 1935) in Stockholm and by Schinz and Zuppinger (1937) in Zürich. On the other hand, the Report of the W.H.O. Expert Committee (1966) favours the 'specialised centre or cancer institute'. It is understood of course, that in other countries, local factors must play an important part in decisions of this type.

(2) *Science as the servant and not the master in the treatment of patients with cancer*

In presenting this view, which I think is self-evident if one accepts the need for 'patient-oriented' individualised treatment, it is important to distinguish clearly between science and the scientists. I certainly regard the physicists, chemists and biologists in the hospitals and laboratories as equal professional members of the team, who often have responsibilities at least as serious as my own, even though the ultimate responsibility for treating the patient must rest with a medically qualified person.

Although we are likely to be influenced to an ever-increasing extent by scientific methods and the results of scientific research we must never forget the human side of the treatment of the patients. Finally, in considering care of patients in hospitals, may I recall what Sir Thomas More said about 'public hospitals' in his Utopia (1516): 'These hospitals are very well furnished and equipped with everything condusive to health. Besides, such tender and careful treatment and such constant attendance of expert physicians are provided that, though no one is sent to them against his will, there is hardly anybody in the whole city who, when suffering from illness, does not prefer to be nursed there rather than at home'. Can we attain this standard today?

REFERENCES

(See also Appendix, p. 124)

I. INTRODUCTION

FORSSELL, G. (1928). On the permanency of radiological healing in malignant tumours. *Acta Radiol.* Suppl. II. P. A. Norstedt & Söner, Stockholm. 83 p.

LAZARUS, P. (1928). Handbuch der gesamten Strahlenheilkunde. Erster Band. Die physikalischen, chemischen und pathologischen Grundlagen der gesamten Strahlenbiologie und-Therapie. 825 p.

LAZARUS, P. (1931). Zweiter Band. Strahlenklinik und spezielle therapeutische Methodik. 1292 p. J. F. Bergmann, München.

MULLER, H. J. (1927). Artificial transmutation of the gene. *Science* **66**, 84.

MULLER, H. J. (1928). The effects of X-radiation on genes and chromosomes. *Science* **67**, 82.

REGAUD, C. (1928). Quelle est la valeur et quels doivent être l'organisation et l'équipement des institutions pour le traitement du cancer par le radium et par les rayons X? *Radiophysiologie et Radiothérapie* (Les Presses Universitaires de France). **1** (II), 135. Report to the International Conference at Lake Mohonk, N.Y., 1926.

A brief introduction to some basic topics (pp. 4–8)

AMBROSE, E. J., JAMES, A. M. & LOWICK, J. H. B. (1956). Differences between the electrical charge carried by normal and homologous tumour cells. *Nature* (Lond.) **177**, 576.

BLOOM, H. J. G. (1950). Prognosis in cancer of the breast. *Brit. J. Cancer* **4**, 259.

BURCH, P. R. J. (1970). New approach to cancer. *Nature* (Lond.) **255**, 512.

CUTLER, S. J., BLACK, M. M., MORK, T., HARVEI, S. & FREEMAN, C. (1969). Further observations on prognostic factors in cancer of the female breast. *Cancer* **24**, 653.

FIDLER, H. K., BOYES, D. A. & WORTH, A. J. (1968). Cervical cancer detection in British Columbia: a progress report. *J. Obstet. Gynaec. Brit. Cmwlth.* **75**, 392.

FISHER, E. R. & FISHER, B. (1967). Recent observations on concepts of metastasis. *Arch. Path.* **83**, 321.

FISHMAN, W. H. (1969). Immunologic and biochemical approaches to alkaline phosphatase isoenzyme analysis; the Regan isoenzyme. *Ann. N.Y. Acad. Sci.* **166,** Art. 2, 745.

GASIC, G. J., GASIC, T. B. & STEWART, C. C. (1968). Antimetastatic effects associated with platelet reduction. *Proc. N.A.S.* **61,** 46.

GILBERTSON, V. A. & WANGENSTEEN, O. H. (1964). Cancer detection studies of the rectum, in International Symposium on End Results of Cancer Therapy. *National Cancer Institute Monograph 15.* Ed. S. J. Cutler. U.S. Government Printing Office, Washington, D.C.; see p. 321.

GOODALL, C. M. (1949). On para-endocrine cancer syndromes; a review. *Int. J. Cancer* **4,** 1.

HAMLIN, I. M. E. (1968). Possible host resistance in carcinoma of the breast; a histological study. *Brit. J. Cancer* **22,** 383.

HARRIS, R. J. C. (Ed.) (1967). Specific Tumour Antigens. *U.I.C.C. Monograph Series,* Vol. 2. Munksgaard, Copenhagen. 366 p.

IVERSEN, O. H. (1967). Kinetics of cellular proliferation and cell loss in human carcinomas. *Europ. J. Cancer* **3,** 389.

KISSEN, D. M. & LESHAN, L. L. (Ed.) (1964) *Psychosomatic aspects of neoplastic disease.* Pitman Medical Publishing Co., London, 231 p.

MCLAREN, H. C. (1963). *The prevention of cervical cancer.* The English Universities Press, London. 134 p.

MEHRISHI, J. N. (1969). Effect of lysine polypeptides on the surface charge of normal and cancer cells. *Europ. J. Cancer* **5,** 427.

MENDELSOHN, M. L. (1965). The kinetics of tumour cell proliferation in *Cellular Radiation Biology.* Williams and Wilkins, Baltimore. p. 498.

MITCHELL, J. S. (1960). *Studies in Radiotherapeutics.* Blackwell Scientific Publications, Oxford and Harvard University Press, Cambridge, Massachussets, see p. 12.

REFSUM, S. B. & BERDAL, P. (1967). Cell loss in malignant tumours in man. *Europ. J. Cancer* **3,** 235.

REGISTRAR GENERAL (1967). The Registrar General's Statistical Review of England and Wales for the Year 1961. *Supplement on Cancer.* H.M.S.O., London, 62 p.

ROSS, E. J. (1968). The cancer cell as an endocrine organ, in *Recent Advances in Endocrinology.* Ed. V. H. Y. James. J. and A. Churchill Ltd, London. 8th Ed. Chap. 10, p. 293.

SIMON-REUSS, I., COOK, G. M. W., SEAMAN, G. V. F. & HEARD, D. H. (1964). Electrophoretic studies on some types of mammalian tissue cell. *Cancer Res.* **24,** 2038.

SMITHERS, D. W. (1962). Cancer, an attack on cytologism. *Lancet* **i,** 443.

STEEL, G. G. (1968). Cell loss from experimental tumours. *Cell Tissue Kinet.* **1,** 193.

TAPTIKLIS, N. (1969). Penetration of the vascular endothelial barrier by non-neoplastic thyroid cells in circulation. *Europ. J. Cancer* **5**, 445.

TUBIANA, M., FRINDEL, E. & MALAISE, E. (1969). *In vivo* cell kinetics of human cancers, in *Normal and malignant cell growth*. Ed. R. J. M. Fry, M. L. Griem and W. H. Kirsten. *Recent Results in Cancer Research 17*. Springer, Berlin, Heidelberg, New York, p. 202.

WIMHÖFER, H., WAGNER, D. & SCHUNK, R. (1963). Der Tumorzellnachweis im strömenden Blut während therapeutischer Massnahmen beim Genitalkarzinom der Frau. *Zentralblatt f. Gynäk.* **85**, 10.

The magnitude of the task (pp. 8–9)

Cancer Records Bureau of the East Anglian Region (1969) *Annual Report 1967–68*. Addenbrooke's Hospital, Cambridge. 19 p.

Chief Medical Officer (1969). On the state of the public health. *The Annual Report of the Chief Medical Officer of the Department of Health and Social Security for the year 1968*. H.M.S.O., London. 276 p.

DOLL, R. (1967) Prevention of cancer. Pointers from epidemiology. The Rock Carling Fellowship. 1967. The Nuffield Provincial Hospital Trust. Whitefriars Press, London, 143 p.

DOLL, R., PAYNE, P. & WATERHOUSE, J. (1966). Cancer incidence in five continents. International Union against Cancer. Springer, Berlin-Heidelberg-New York. 244 p.

DUNHAM, L. J. & BAILAR, J. C. (1968). World maps of cancer mortality rates and frequency ratios. *J. Nat. Cancer Inst.* **41**, 155.

World Health Organization (1966). Cancer Treatment. Report of a WHO Expert Committee. *WHO Technical Report Series* No. 322. WHO, Geneva, see p. 50.

A discussion of methods of treatment (pp. 9–19)

BAGSHAWE, K. D. (1969). *Choriocarcinoma. The clinical biology of the trophoblast and its tumours*. Edward Arnold, London. 360 p.

BROERSE, J. J. & BARENDSEN, G. W. (1970). Measurments of absorbed doses due to exposure of organs of different composition to fast neutrons of different energies. Euratom Report: EUR 4465e.

CLARK, R. LEE (Ed.) (1961). *Cancer Chemotherapy*. Charles C. Thomas, Springfield, Illinois, U.S.A. 253 p.

COBB, J. P., WALKER, D. G. and WRIGHT, J. C. (1961). Comparative chemotherapy studies on primary short-term cultures of human normal, benign and malignant tumour tissues – a five year study. *Cancer Res.* **21**, 583.

COHEN, L. & SCOTT, M. J. (1968). Fractionation procedures in radiation therapy: a computerised approach to evaluation. *Brit. J. Radiol.* **41**, 529.

DENDY, P. P. (1968) Responses of freshly cultured tumour cells to certain selected chemotherapeutic agents. *J. Obst. Gyn. Brit. Comwth.* **75**, 1256.

DENDY, P. P., BOZMAN, G. & WHEELER, T. K. (1970) *In vitro* screening test for human malignant tumours before chemotherapy. *Lancet* **ii**, 68.

DOGLIOTTI, A. M. (1936). Trattamento del dolore nei tumori. Travaux scientifiques. Tome 1. Rapports généraux. IIe Congres international de lutte scientifique et sociale contre le cancer. Édition: Ligue Nationale belge contre le cancer. Bruxelles. p. 309.

DUNWORTH, J. V. & MITCHELL, J. S. (1945). *Application of nuclear physics to medicine and biology*, 26 March 1945, and *Notes on the preparation of radioactive isotopes for use in medicine and biology*, 17 October 1945. Reports to the Montreal Laboratory of the National Research Council, Canada.

EASSON, E. C. & RUSSELL, M. H. (1968). *The curability of cancer in various sites*. 4th Statistical Report of the Christie Hospital and Holt Radium Institute, Manchester. Pitman Medical Publ. Co., London. 149 p.

ELLIS, F. (1967). Fractionation in radiotherapy, in *Modern Trends in Radiotherapy*, Vol. 1. Ed. T. J. Deeley and C. A. P. Wood, Butterworths, London. Chap. 2, p. 34.

FALKMER, S., FORS, B., LARSSON, B., LINDELL, A., NAESLUND, J. & STENSON, S. (1962). Pilot study on proton irradiation of human carcinoma. *Acta Radiol.* (Stockh.) **58**, 33.

FARBER, S., DIAMOND, L. K., MERCER, R. D., SYLVESTER, R. F. & WOLFF, J. A. (1948). Temporary remissions in acute leukaemia in children produced by folic acid antagonist, 4-aminopteroylglutamic acid (aminopterin). *New England J. Med.* **238**, 787.

FARR, L. E., SWEET, W. H., ROBERTSON, J. S., FOSTER, C. G., LOCKSLEY, H. B., SUTHERLAND, D. L., MENDELSOHN, M. L. & STICKLEY, E. E. (1954). Neutron capture therapy with Boron in the treatment of glioblastoma multiforme. *Amer. J. Roentgenol.* **71**, 279.

FOWLER, J. F. (1967). Fast neutron therapy – physical and biological considerations, in *Modern Trends in Radiotherapy*, Vol. 1. Ed. T. J. Deeley and C. A. P. Wood. Butterworths, London. Chap. 8, p. 145.

FOWLER, P. H. & PERKINS, D. H. (1961). The possibility of therapeutic applications of beams of negative Pi-mesons. *Nature* (Lond.) **189**, 524.

FREUNDLICH, H. F., HAYBITTLE, J. L. & QUICK, R. S. (1950). Radioiridium teletherapy. *Acta Radiol.* (Stockh.) **34**, 115.

GRAFFMAN, S. & JUNG, B. (1970). Clinical trials in radiotherapy and the merits of high energy protons. *Acta Radiol. Ther. Phys. Biol.* **9**, 1.

HADDOW, A. & SEXTON, W. A. (1946). Influence of carbamic esters (urethanes) on experimental animal tumours. *Nature* (Lond.) **157**, 500.

HALL, E. J. (1969). Time dose and fractionation in radiotherapy; a comparison of two evaluation systems in clinical use. *Brit. J. Radiol.* **42**, 427.

HALL, E. J., BEDFORD, J. S. & OLIVER, R. (1966). Extreme hypoxia; its effect on the survival of mammalian cells irradiated at high and low dose-rates. *Brit. J. Radiol.* **39**, 302.

HAYBITTLE, J. L. (1964). A 24-curie strontium-90 unit for whole-body superficial irradiation with beta-rays. *Brit. J. Radiol.* **37**, 297.

HAYBITTLE, J. L. & DALLISON, J. (1958). A caesium^{137} gamma-ray therapy unit. *Acta Radiol.* (Stockh.) **50**, 321.

HAYBITTLE, J. L. & HOUSTON, A. A. (1968). The use of a multi-access computer for radiation treatment planning. *Brit. J. Radiol.* **41**, 927.

HERTZ, R. (1967). In *Choriocarcinoma*. Ed. J. F. Holland and Hreshchyskyn, M. M. *U.I.C.C. Monograph Series*, Vol. 3. Springer, Berlin, Heidelberg, New York. p. 66.

HERTZ, R., BERGENSTAL, D. M., LIPSETT, M. B., PRICE, E. B. and HILBISH, T. F. (1958). Chemotherapy of choriocarcinoma and related trophoblastic tumours in women. *J. Amer. med. Ass.* **168**, 845.

HORWITZ, H. & HAYBITTLE, J. L. (1960). Whole body superficial irradiation with strontium 90 beta rays. A report of cases treated with a moving couch technique. *Brit. J. Radiol.* **33**, 440.

International Atomic Energy Agency (1968). *Directory of high-energy radiotherapy centres.* STI/PUBI/77, IAEA, Vienna, 189 p.

JANTET, GEORGES. (1969). Intralymphatic therapy, Chap. 11 in *Lymphography in Cancer*. Ed. W. A. Fuchs, J. W. Davidson, H. W. Fischer, *Recent Results in Cancer Research 23*. William Heinemann Medical Books, London; Springer, Berlin, Heidelberg, New York, p. 265.

KAPLAN, H. S. (1966). Long-term results of palliative and radical radiotherapy of Hodgkin's disease. *Cancer Res.* **26**, 1250.

KARNOFSKY, D. A. (1964). Chemotherapy of cancer and its present position in the management of neoplastic disease, in *Chemotherapy of Cancer*, Ed. P. A. Plattner. Elsevier, Amsterdam, London, New York, p. 3.

KARRER, K. (1964). Zur kombinierten cytostatischen und operativen Behandlung des Carcinoma. *Arzneimittel-Forschung* **14**, 859 and 1059.

KJELLBERG, R. N., SWEET, W. H., PRESTON, W. M. & KOEHLER, A. M. (1962). The Bragg peak of a proton beam in intracranial therapy of tumours. *Trans. Amer. neurol. Ass.* **87**, 216.

LACHER, M. J. (1969). Long survival in Hodgkin's disease. *Ann. Intern. Med.* **70**, 7.

LAWRENCE, J. H. & TOBIAS, C. A. (1967). Heavy particles in therapy, in *Modern Trends in Radiotherapy*, Vol. 1. Ed. T. J. Deeley and C. A. P. Wood. Butterworths, London. Chap. 15, p. 260.

LEDERMAN, M. (1953). Radiotherapy of epibulbar malignant melanomata. *Trans. Ophthal. Soc.* **73**, 399.

LEDERMAN, M. (1956). Some applications of radioactive isotopes in ophthalmology. *Brit. J. Radiol.* **29**, 1.

LIMBURG, H. & HECKMANN, U. (1968). Chemotherapy in the treatment of advanced pelvic malignant disease with special reference to ovarian cancer. *J. Obstet. Gyn. Br. Cmwlth.* **75**, 1246.

LIMBURG, H. & KRAHE, M. (1964). Die Züchtung von menschlichem Krebsgewebe in der Gewebekultur und seine Sensibilitätstestung gegen neuere Zytostatika. *Dtsch. med. Wschr.* **89**, 1938.

MAEDA, M. & SUIT, H. D. (1965). Radiation dose fractionation and oxygen effect in a mammary carcinoma of the C3H mouse. Comm. at XIth Int. Congr. of Radiology, Rome, Int. Congr. series 89 Excerpta Medica Foundation, Abstr. No. 980.

Medical Research Council's Working Party for Therapeutic Trials in Leukaemia (1968). Chronic granulocytic leukaemia: comparison of radiotherapy and bisulphan therapy. *Brit. med. J.* **1**, 201.

MITCHELL, J. S. (1946). Applications of recent advances in nuclear physics to medicine. *Brit. J. Radiol.* **19**, 481.

MITCHELL, J. S. (1960). *Studies in Radiotherapeutics.* Blackwell Scientific Publications, Oxford and Harvard University Press, Cambridge, Massachusetts, see p. 200.

MITCHELL, J. S. (1968). Applied science and the development of radiotherapy – past, present and future. *Brit. J. Radiol.* **41**, 729.

MITCHELL, J. S. & MITCHELL, L. M. (1967). Fractionation in radiotherapy of cancer of the lip. *Acta radiol. Ther. Phys. Biol.* **6**, 299.

MITCHELL, J. S. & STERLING, T. D. (Chairmen) (1967). *The use of computers in therapeutic radiology.* Summary Report of an International Conference held in Cambridge, England, 14–17 June 1966. British Institute of Radiology, 32 Welbeck Street, London, W.1. 29 p.

MORE, SIR THOMAS (1516). *Utopia*; see The Yale Edition. Ed. E. Surtz (1964). Yale University Press, New Haven and London. See p. 108.

MORGAN, R. L. (1967). Fast neutron therapy – clinical applications, in *Modern Trends in Radiotherapy*, Vol. 1. Ed. T. J. Deeley and C. A. P. Wood. Butterworths, London, Chap. 9, p. 171.

MORGAN, R. L. (1968). Neutron therapy. *Ann. Rep. Brit. Emp. Cancer Campaign for Research*, p. 90.

MÜLLER, J. H. (1961). *Interne Tumortherapie mit künstlich radioaktiven Isotopen.* (Exclusive Blutkrankheiten und Schilddrüse) in Künstliche Radioaktive Isotope in Physiologie, Diagnostik und Therapie, 2 Aufl. Bd. II, Hrsg. H. Schwiegk u. F. Turba, Springer, Berlin, Göttingen, Heidelberg, S. 50.

MUNDINGER, F. (1969). Die intraselläre protrahierte Langzeitbestrahlung von Hypophysenadenomen mittels stereotaktischer Implantation von Iridium 192. *Acta radiol. Ther. Phys. Biol.* **8**, 55.

REFERENCES

MUNDINGER, F. (1969). Technik und Indikationen der interstitiellen Bestrahlung mit Radionukliden bei Hirn- und Hypophysengeschwülsten; Techniques and indications for the interstitial irradiation of brain and pituitary tumours with radionuclides. *Kerntechnik* **11**, 333.

OATES, G. D. (1968). Sensitivities of human tumours to chemotherapeutic agents *in vitro*. *Ann. Rep. Brit. Emp. Cancer Campaign for Research*, p. 257.

PETERS, M. V. (1950). A study of survivals in Hodgkin's disease treated radiologically. *Amer. J. Roentgen.* **63**, 299.

PILLERS, E. M. Kingsley (1955). *The sternal bone marrow in malignancy.* M.D. Thesis, University of Cambridge.

PILLERS, E. M. Kinglsey (1965). The bone marrow as a guide to prognosis and treatment of malignant disease, in *The Treatment of Cancer with special reference to radiotherapy and chemotherapy*. Ed. J. S. Mitchell. The University Press, Cambridge, p. 89.

PILLERS, E. M. Kingsley, MARKS, J. & MITCHELL, J. S. (1956). The bone marrow in malignant disease. *Brit. J. Cancer* **10**, 458.

PUCK, T. T. & MARCUS, P. I. (1956). Action of X-rays on single mammalian cells. *J. Exp. Med.* **103**, 653.

PUCK, T. T., MARCUS, P. I. & CIECIURA, S. J. (1956). Clonal growth of mammalian cells *in vitro*. *J. Exp. Med.* **103**, 273.

The Radiochemical Centre, Amersham, Buckinghamshire (1970). Personal communication.

SAMBROOK, D. K. (1968). Further experience with split-course radiotherapy, in *Front. Radiat. Ther. Oncol.* Vol. 3. Karger, Basel and New York, p. 180.

SMITHERS, D. W. (1969). Factors influencing survival in patients with Hodgkin's disease. *Clin. Radiol.* **20**, 124.

STRANDQUIST, M. (1944). Studien über die kumulative Wirkung der Röntgenstrahlen bei Fraktionierung. *Acta radiol. Stockh. Suppl* 55.

THOMLINSON, R. H. (1966). *The effects of irradiation on the proportion of anoxic cells in tumours.* Communication at Third Inst. Congr. of Radiation Research, Cortina d'Ampezzo, Abstr. No. 878.

TSIEN, K. C. (1955). The application of automatic computing machines to radiation treatment planning. *Brit. J. Radiol.* **28**, 432.

VAN PUTTEN, L. M. (1968). Tumour reoxygenation during fractionated radiotherapy; studies with a transplantable mouse osteosarcoma. *Europ. J. Cancer* **4**, 173–182.

VAN PUTTEN, L. M. & KALLMAN, R. F. (1968). Oxygenation status of a transplantable tumour during fractionated radiation therapy. *J. Nat. Cancer Inst.* **40**, 441–451.

WILKES, E. (1970). The family doctor in cancer care, in *People and Cancer*. Ed. G. Bennette. British Cancer Council, 2, Harley Street, London, p. 31.

WRIGHT, C. N., BOULOGNE, A. R., REINIG, W. C. & EVANS, A. G. (1967). Implantable californium-252 neutron sources for radiotherapy. *Radiology* **89**, 337.

YOUNGMAN, H. R. (1965). The treatment of pain by nerve blocking, in *The Treatment of Cancer*. Ed. J. S. Mitchell. The University Press, Cambridge, p. 154.

II. ASSESSMENT OF THE RESULTS OF TREATMENT (pp. 20–23)

Cancer Records Bureau of the East Anglian Region, Addenbrooke's Hospital, Cambridge (1969). *Annual Report, year 1967–68*. Board of Governors, United Cambridge Hospitals and East Anglian Regional Hospital Board, Cambridge. 19 p.

Cancer Records Bureau, South Western Regional Hospital Board (1968). *Annual Report No. 15*, South Western Regional Hospital Board, Dove Lane, Bristol, 2. 55 p.

CUTLER, S. J. (Ed.) (1964). International symposium on end results of cancer therapy. *National Cancer Institute Monograph 15*. U.S. Gov. Printing Office, Washington, D.C., 446 p.

HARNETT, W. L. (1952). A survey of cancer in London. *Report of the Clinical Research Committee, British Empire Cancer Campaign*. London. 834 p.

KARNOFSKY, D. A., BURCHENAL. J. H., ARMISTEAD, G. C., SOUTHAM, C. M., BERNSTEIN, J. L., CRAVER, L. F. & RHOADS, C. P. (1951). Triethylene melamine in the treatment of neoplastic disease. *A.M.A. Arch. int. Med.* **87**, 477.

NYSTRÖM, G. (1922). Kräftsjukdomarne i Sverige. *Svenska Cancerföreningen*, Stockholm. 400 p.

REGISTRAR GENERAL (1967). The Registrar General's Statistical Review of England and Wales for the year 1961: *Supplement on Cancer*. General Register Office. H.M.S.O., London. 62 p.

The cured group (pp. 23–26)

BELONOSCHKIN, B. (1955). Das Auftreten des Karzinoms nach der 5-jährigen Heilungsdauer des bestrahlten Carcinoma Colli Uteri. *Acta Radiol.* (Stockh.) **44**, 57.

BERKSON, J. & GAGE, R. P. (1952). Survival curve for cancer patients following treatment. *J. Amer. Statistical Ass.* **47**, 501.

BLOOM, H. J. G., WALLACE, E. N. K. & HENK, J. M. (1969). The treatment and prognosis of medulloblastoma in children. *Amer. J. Roentgenol.* **105**, 43.

BOAG, J. W. (1948). The presentation and analysis of the results of radiotherapy. *Brit. J. Radiol.* **21**, 128 and 189.

BOAG, J. W. (1949). Maximum likelihood estimates of the proportion of patients cured by cancer therapy. *J. Roy. Statist. Soc.* Series B, **XI,** 1, 15.

BOND, W. H. (1968). The influence of various treatments on survival rates in cancer of the breast, in *The Treatment of Carcinoma of the Breast.* Ed. A. S. Jarrett. Publ. for Syntex Pharmaceuticals Ltd by Excepta Medica Foundation. p. 24.

BRINKLEY, D. & HAYBITTLE, J. L. (1968). A 15-year follow-up study of patients treated for carcinoma of the breast. *Brit. J. Radiol.* **41,** 215.

COLLINS, V. P. (1968). The treatment of Wilms's tumour. *Cancer* **11,** 89.

COLLINS, V. P., LOEFFLER, R. K. & TIVEY, H. (1956). Observations on growth rates of human tumours. *Amer. J. Roentgenol.* **76,** 988.

CUTLER, S. J. & AXTELL, L. M. (1963). Partitioning of a patient population with respect to different mortality risks. *J. Amer. Statistical Ass.* **58,** 701.

GREENWOOD, M. (1926). The natural duration of cancer. *Ministry of Health, Reports on Public Health and Medical Subjects,* No. 33. H.M.S.O., London. 26 p.

HAYBITTLE, J. L. (1959). The estimation of the proportion of patients cured after treatment for cancer of the breast. *Brit. J. Radiol.* **32,** 725.

HAYBITTLE, J. L. (1960). The early estimation of the results of treatment for cancer. *Brit. J. Radiol.* **33,** 502.

HAYBITTLE, J. L. (1964). The cured group in series of patients treated for cancer. *Anglo-German Medical Review* (Stuttgart) **2,** 422.

KNOX, W. E. & KINGSLEY PILLERS, E. M. (1958). Time of recurrence or cure of tumours in childhood. *Lancet* **i,** 188.

KOTTMEIER, H.-L. (1962). Ten year end results, radiological treatment of carcinoma of the cervix. *Acta obst. et gynec. scandinav.* **41,** 195.

KOTTMEIER, H.-L. & FORSSNER, E. (1955). Die Entwicklung der Therapie des Kollumkarzinoms am Radiumhemmet. *München. med. Wschr.* **97,** 1019.

MARSDEN, H. B. & STEWARD, J. K. (Ed.) (1968). Tumours in Children. *Recent Results in Cancer Research 13.* Springer, Berlin, Heidelberg, New York. see p. 245.

Investigation of new methods of treatment (pp. 26–28)

ABBÉ, T. (1904). Notes on the physiologic and the therapeutic action of radium. *Washington Med. Ann.* **2,** 363.

DEUTSCH, J. (1904). Die Radiotherapie bei Gebärmutter-geschwülsten. *München. med. Wschr.* 1646.

DÖDERLEIN, A. (1913). Verh. des Kongresses der Deutschen Gesellschaft für Gynäkologie, Halle a.d. Saale. See also

DÖDERLEIN, A. (1938). Die Entdeckung des Radiums und der radioaktiven Substanzen in ihrer Bedeutung für die Behandlung des Uteruskarzinoms. *Strahlentherapie* **63,** 403.

FORSSELL, G. (1928). On the permanency of radiological healing in malignant tumours. *Acta Radiol.* Suppl. II. P. A. Norstedt & Söner, Stockholm, see p. 30.

KOTTMEIER, H.-L. (1967). Annual report on the results of treatment in carcinoma of the uterus and vagina. Norstedt, Stockholm.

RIES, J. & BREITNER, J. (1959). Strahlenbehandlung in der Gynäkologie. Sonderbände zur Strahlentherapie, Bd. 40. Urban und Schwarzenberg, München, Berlin. 219S.

Clinical trials (pp. 28–36)

ARMITAGE, P. (1954). Sequential tests in prophylactic and therapeutic trials. *Quart. J. Med.* **23**, 255.

ARMITAGE, P. (1960). *Sequential Medical Trials.* Blackwell Scientific Publications, Oxford. 105 p.

BANKIER, J. D. & BATLEY, F. (1957). Comparative series in evaluation of cancer therapy. *Brit. J. Radiol.* **30**, 158.

BOAG, J. W. (1948). The presentation and analysis of the results of radiotherapy. *Brit. J. Radiol.* **21**, 128 and 189.

BOAG, J. W. (1960). Statistical problems which arise in cancer therapy. *Clin. Radiol.* **11**, 150.

BOND, W. H. (1970). The prognostic implication of treatment. *Proc. Soc. Roy. Med.* **63**, 111.

BRINKLEY, D. & HAYBITTLE, J. L. (1959). Results of treatment of carcinoma of the breast. *Lancet* **i**, 86.

BRINKLEY, D. & HAYBITTLE, J. L. (1965). Some aspects of clinical trials, in *The Treatment of Cancer*. Ed. J. S. Mitchell. The University Press, Cambridge. p. 135.

BRINKLEY, D. & HAYBITTLE, J. L. (1966). Treatment of stage-II carcinoma of the female breast. *Lancet* **ii**, 291.

BROSS, I. (1952). Sequential medical plans. *Biometrics* **8**, 188.

Declaration of Helsinki (Code of Ethics of the World Medical Association) (1964). *Brit. med. J.* **i**, 177.

DEELEY, T. J. (1967). Controlled clinical trials in radiotherapy, in *Modern Trends in Radiotherapy*, Vol. 1. Ed. T. J. Deeley and C. A. P. Wood. Butterworths, London, Chap. 11, p. 208.

EASSON, E. C. (1968). Post-operative radiotherapy in breast cancer, in *Prognostic Factors in Breast Cancer*. Ed. A. P. M. Forrest and P. B. Kunkler. E. and S. Livingstone, Edinburgh and London, p. 118.

FISHER, R. A. (1925). *Statistical methods for research workers.* Oliver and Boyd, Edinburgh. 356 p.

FISHER, R. A. (1935). *The design of experiments.* Oliver and Boyd, Edinburgh and London. 6th Ed., 1951. 244 p.

GEHAN, E. A. (1961). The determination of the number of patients required in a preliminary and a follow-up trial of a new chemotherapeutic agent. *J. Chron. Dis.* **13**, 346.

GRAFFMAN, S. & JUNG, B. (1970). Clinical trials in radiotherapy and the merits of high energy protons. *Acta radiol. Ther. Phys. Biol.* **9**, 1.

HALSTED, W. S. (1894). Results of operation for cure of cancer of breast performed at Johns Hopkins Hospital from June 1889 to January 1894. *Ann. Surgery* **20**, 497.

HEALEY, J. & ANDERSON, F. (1965). Cytotoxic drugs in bronchial carcinoma. *Lancet* **i**, 1119.

HILL, A. Bradford (1970). The power and limitations of statistical methods, in *People and cancer*, and *The problem of relevance in cancer research*. Ed. G. Bennette. The British Cancer Council, 2, Harley Street, London, p. 79, see p. 81.

KAAE, S. & JOHANSEN, H. (1965). In *Progress in clinical cancer*, Vol. 1. Ed. I. M. Ariel. Grune and Stratton, New York, p. 453.

KAAE, S. & JOHANSEN, H. (1968). Simple versus radical mastectomy in primary breast cancer, in *Prognostic factors in breast cancer*. Ed. A. P. M. Forrest and P. B. Kunkler. E. and S. Livingstone, Edinburgh and London. p. 93.

KARNOFSKY, D. A., BURCHENAL, J. H., ARMISTEAD, G. C., SOUTHAM, C. M., BERNSTEIN, J. L., CRAVER, L. F. & RHOADS, C. P. (1951). Triethylene melamine in the treatment of neoplastic disease. *A.M.A. Arch. int. Med.* **87**, 477.

KAUFMANN, H. (1969). Allgemeine Gesichtspunkte zur Darstellung von Behandlungsergebnissen bei tödlich verlaufenden Erkrankungen. *Strahlentherapie* **130**, 81.

KAUFMANN, H. (1966). Ein einfaches Verfahren zur Auswertung von Überlebenskurven bei tödlich verlaufenden Erkrankungen. *Strahlentherapie* **130**, 509.

Lancet (1969). Treatment of early cancer of the breast. **ii**, 1175.

LEE, BURTON, J. (1928). Conservatism in the treatment of primary operable cancer of the breast. Five-year results in 73 cases, treated by irradiation alone, or in conjunction with conservative surgery. *Report of the International Conference on Cancer, London 17–20 July, 1928. Brit. Emp. Cancer Campaign*, London, p. 131.

LENARDUZZI, G., VALDAGNI, C. & PISTOLESI, G. F. (1965). Comparison of the results of treatment of 2,549 cases of malignant neoplasm with high-energy radiation in *Progress in Radiology*, Proc. XI Intern. Congr. Radiology, Rome (cit. Graffman and Jung, 1970).

MARRIAN, D. H., MARSHALL, B. & MITCHELL, J. S. (1961). Laboratory and clinical studies of some quinol diphosphates and related compounds as chemical radiosensitizers and the development of a radioactive drug. *Chemotherapia* **3**, 225; see pp. 254, 262.

MCWHIRTER, R. (1955). Simple mastectomy and radiotherapy in the treatment of breast cancer. *Brit. J. Radiol.* **28**, 128.

Medical Research Council (1948). Streptomycin treatment of pulmonary tuberculosis. *Brit. med. J.* **ii**, 769.

Medical Research Council (1950). Treatment of pulmonary tuberculosis with streptomycin and para-amino-salicylic acid. *Brit. med. J.* **ii,** 1073.

Medical Research Council (1964). Responsibility in investigation on human subjects. *Brit. med. J.* **i,** 178.

MITCHELL, J. S. (1960). *Studies in Radiotherapeutics.* Blackwell Scientific Publications, Oxford, and Harvard University Press, Cambridge, Massachusetts. See pp. 137, 140, 160.

MITCHELL, J. S. (1965). An attempt to develop a radioactive drug. *Clin. Radiol.* **14,** 305.

MITCHELL, J. S., BRINKLEY, D. & HAYBITTLE, J. L. (1965). Clinical trial of radiosensitizers, including Synkavit and oxygen inhaled at atmospheric pressure. *Acta Radiol. Ther. Phys. Biol.* **3,** 329.

PAPPWORTH, M. H. (1967). *Human guinea pigs, Experimentation on man.* Routledge and Kegan Paul, London. 228 p.

PATNAIK, P. B. (1948). The power function of the test for the difference between two proportions in a 2 × 2 table. *Biometrika* **35,** 157.

WALD, A. (1947). *Sequential Analysis.* Wiley, New York.

WRIGHTON, R. F. (1953). The theoretical basis of the therapeutic trial. *Acta Genetica et Statistica Medica* **4,** 312.

III. DEVELOPMENT OF RESEARCH IN RELATION TO RADIOTHERAPY (pp. 37–39)

BIRDSALL, N. J. M. (1967). *Synthesis and distribution studies of two tritiated ubiquinone derivatives.* Ph.D. Dissertation, University of Cambridge.

MITCHELL, J. S. (1940). Increase in ultra-violet absorption of cytoplasm after therapeutic X- and gamma-irradiation, *Nature* (Lond.) **146,** 272.

MITCHELL, J. S. (1942). Disturbance of nucleic acid metabolism produced by therapeutic doses of X- and gamma-radiations. Part 1. Methods of investigation. *Brit. J. Exp. Path.* **23,** 285.

MITCHELL, J. S. (1942). Disturbance of nucleic acid metabolism produced by therapeutic doses of X- and gamma-radiations. Part 2. Accumulation of pentose nucleotides in cytoplasm after irradiation. *Brit. J. Exp. Path.* **23,** 296.

MITCHELL, J. S. (1942). Disturabnce of nucleic acid metabolism produced by doses of X- and gamma-radiations. Part 3. Inhibition of synthesis of thymonucleic acid by radiation. *Brit. J. Exp. Path.* **23,** 309.

MITCHELL, J. S. (1942). Medical uses of radium: measurement of the effects of X- and gamma-irradiation on normal and malignant cells by means of ultra-violet photomicrography. *Brit. J. Radiol.* **15,** 59.

Mitchell, J. S. (1943). Metabolic effects of therapeutic doses of X- and gamma-radiations. *Brit. J. Radiol.* **16,** 339.

Mitchell, J. S. (1944). Disturbance of nucleic acid metabolism produced by therapeutic doses of X- and gamma-radiations. *Brit. Empire Cancer Campaign, 21st Annual Report,* p. 62.

Mitchell, J. S. (1948). Clinical trials of tetra-sodium 2-methyl-1:4-naphthohydroquinone diphosphate, in conjunction with X-ray therapy. *Brit. J. Cancer* **2,** 351.

Mitchell, J. S. (1956). Some problems of radiotherapeutics. *Proceedings of the International Conference on the Peaceful Uses of Atomic Energy,* 1955, Geneva, **10,** 25. United Nations: New York.

Mitchell, J. S. (1956). The 'macromolecular lesion' involving deoxyribonucleic acid in radiobiology and radiotherapy. *J. Colloid Science* **11,** 317.

Mitchell, J. S. (1960). *Studies in Radiotherapeutics,* Blackwell Scientific Publications, Oxford, and Harvard University Press, Cambridge, Massachusetts. 274 p.

Mitchell, J. S. & Simon-Reuss, I. (1952). Experiments on the mechanism of action of tetra-sodium 2-methyl-1:4-naphthohydroquinone diphosphate as a mitotic inhibitor and radiosensitiser, using the technique of tissue culture. Experimental methods and quantitative results. *Brit. J. Cancer* **6,** 305.

Mitchell, J. S. & Simon-Reuss, I. (1952). Experiments on the mechanism of action of tetra-sodium 2-methyl-1:4-naphthohydroquinone diphosphate as a mitotic inhibitor and radiosensitiser, using the technique of tissue culture. Relation between cytological effects and chemical constitution. *Brit. J. Cancer* **6,** 317.

Young, J. M. (1963). *Studies on two potential tritiated drugs.* Ph.D. Dissertation, University of Cambridge.

Young, J. M., Wild, F. & Simon-Reuss, I. (1965). Studies of the uptake of tritium labelled mepacrine by tumours. *Brit. J. Cancer* **19,** 370.

Radiosensitizers (pp. 39–50)

Adams, G. E. (1967). The general application of pulse radiolysis to current problems in radiobiology, in *Topics in Radiation Research,* Vol. III. Ed. M. Ebert and A. Howard. North-Holland Publ., Amsterdam, p. 35.

Adams, G. E. (1968). Pulse radiolysis in radiobiology: Some recent studies on model systems, in *Radiation Chemistry of Aqueous Systems.* Ed. G. Stein. The Weizman Press of Israel, Jerusalem. John Wiley and Sons, London, New York ,Sydney, p. 241.

Adams, G. E. & Cooke, M. S. (1969). Electron-affinic sensitization. 1. A structural basis for chemical radiosensitizers in bacteria. *Int. J. Rad. Biol.* **15,** 457.

ADAMS, G. E., COOKE, M. S. & MICHAEL, B. D. (1968). Rapid mixing in radiobiology. *Nature* (Lond.) **219,** 1368.

ADAMS, G. E. & DEWEY, D. L. (1963). Hydrated electrons and radiobiological sensitization. *Biochem. biophys. Res. Commun.* **12,** 473.

ASHWOOD-SMITH, M. J., ROBINSON, D. M., BARNES, J. H. & BRIDGES, B. A. (1967). Radiosensitization of bacterial and mammalian cells by substituted glyoxals. *Nature* **216,** 137.

BARNES, J. H., ASHWOOD-SMITH, M. J. & BRIDGES, B. A. (1969). Radiosensitization of bacterial cells by carboxyl compounds. *Int. J. Radiat. Biol.* **15,** 285.

BECKER, H. W. (1965). Klinische Untersuchungen über den Einfluss von Vitamin K_3 auf das Bronchialkarzinom unter Strahlentherapie. *Rad. biol. ther.* **6**/2, 285.

BEGG, A. C., DENEKAMP, J. & HOWES, A. E. (1969). Re-oxygenation of tumours after irradiation and cell population kinetics. *Proc. Physiol. Soc.*, Feb. 1969, D.11. 16 P.

BIRDSALL, N. J. M. (1967). *Synthesis and distribution studies of two tritiated ubiquinone derivatives.* Ph.D. Dissertation, University of Cambridge.

BRIDGES, B. A. (1969). Sensitization of organisms to radiation by sulfhydryl-binding agents. *Adv. in Radiation. Biology*, Vol 3. Academic Press, New York, p. 123.

CHIPPERFIELD, B. (1966). Ubiquinone concentrations in tumours and some normal tissues in man; increased ubiquinone concentrations in tissues of tumour-bearing rats. *Nature* (Lond.) **209,** 1207, 1208.

CHIPPERFIELD, B. & MARRIAN, D. H. (1962). Studies of potential radiosensitizing agents. The effects of 2-methyl-1:4-naphthohydroquinone diphosphate (Synkavit) on the level of adenosine triphosphate in mouse ascites tumour. *Brit. J. Cancer* **16,** 460.

COX, R. P. & GRIFFIN, M. J. (1967). Alkaline phosphatase. I. Comparison of the physical and chemical properties of enzyme preparations from mammalian cell cultures, various animal tissues and Escherichia coli. *Arch. Biochem. Biophys.* **122,** 552.

CRABTREE, H. G. & CRAMER, W. (1933). The action of radium on cancer cells. II. Some factors determining the susceptibility of cancer cells to radium. *Proc. Roy. Soc. B.* **113,** 238.

CRABTREE, H. G. & CRAMER, W. (1934). *11th Sci. Rep. Imp. Cancer Res. Fund*, p. 89.

DEELEY, T. J. (1967). The treatment of carcinoma of the bronchus. *Brit. J. Radiol.* **40,** 801.

DENDY, P. P. (1967) and (1970). Personal communications.

DENDY, P. P. (1969). Selective uptake of a radioactive drug into human tumour cells growing in tissue culture. *Acta Radiol. Ther. Phys. Biol.* **8,** 514.

REFERENCES

DiVita, G. & Marrian, D. H. (1970). Indantrione, menadione, Synkavit and N-ethylmaleimide tested as radiosensitizers on murine ascitic tumour irradiated *in vitro* and grown *in vivo*. *Radiation Protection and sensitization*. Ed. H. Moroson and M. Quintiliani. Taylor and Francis, London, p. 225.

Djordjevic, B. & Szybalski, W. (1960) Genetics of human line cells. III. Incorporation of 5-bromo- and 5-iododeoxyuridine into the deoxyribonucleic acid of human cells and its effects on radiation sensitivity. *J. exp. Med.* **112**, 509.

Doggett, R. L. Scotte, Bagshaw, M. A. & Kaplan, H. S. (1967). Combined therapy using chemotherapeutic agents and radiotherapy in *Modern Trends in Radiotherapy*, Vol. 1. Ed. T. J. Deeley and C. A. P. Wood. Butterworths, London, Chap. 6, p. 107.

Eichhorn, H. J. & Lessel, A. (1968). Spätresultate nach Telekobalttherapie bei histologisch gesichertem, inoperablem Bronchialkarzinom. *Strahlentherapie* **136**, 411.

Eldjarn, L. & Pihl, A. (1960). Mechanisms of protective and sensitizing action, in *Mechanisms in Radiobiology*, Vol. 2. Ed. M. Errera and A. Forssberg. Academic Press, New York. Chap. 4, p. 231.

Evans, C. M. & Todd, I. D. H. (1969). Synkavit and radiotherapy in the treatment of bronchial carcinoma. A random trial. *Clin. Radiol.* **20**, 228.

Fischer Wasels, B. (1930). *Die Gasbehandlung bösartiger Geschwülste*. Frankfurt a.M.

Fisher, V. (1968). Personal communication.

Flemming, K., Mehrishi, J. N. & Napier, J. A. F. (1968). The loss of intracellular K^+ ions from the intact Ehrlich ascites carcinoma cell following irradiation with 15 MeV electrons and X-rays. *Int. J. Radiat. Biol.* **14**, 175.

Foye, W. O. (1967). Anti-radiation Agents. In *Annual Reports in Medicinal Chemistry*, 1966, Chap. 32, p. 330.

Friedmann, E., Marrian, D. H. & Simon-Reuss, I. (1948). Sulphydryl addition compounds of some quinones and related substances in their action on the growth of normal cells. *Brit. J. Pharmacol. Chemother.* **3**, 335.

Galeotti, T., Azzi, A. & Chance, B. (1970). The reoxidation of cytoplasmic reducing equivalents in Ehrlich ascites tumor cells. *Biochim. Biophys. Acta* **197**, 11.

Gellé, X. & Leguerinais, J. (1964). Lung cancer – evaluation of end results in International Symposium of End Results of Cancer Therapy. Ed. S. J. Cutler, *National Cancer Institute Monograph 15*. U.S. Gov. Printing Office, Washington, D.C. p. 37; see p. 39.

Gordon, E. E., Ernster, L. & Dallner, G. (1967). Intracellular hydrogen transport in Ehrlich ascites tumor cells. *Cancer Res.* **27**, 1372.

GÖRÖG, P. & KOVÁCS, I. B. (1967). Effects of vitamins K_1 and K_3 on adenosine nucleotide content of rat tissues. *Molec. Pharmacol.* **3**, 495.

GRAY, L. H. (1957). Oxygenation in radiotherapy. I. Radiobiological considerations. *Brit. J. Radiol.* **30**, 403.

GRONOW, M. (1963). *Synthesis of a radioactive drug and some aspects of its metabolism in tumour cells.* Ph.D. Dissertation, University of Cambridge.

GRONOW, M. (1966). Experiments on the mechanism of the radiosensitization of cells by 2-methyl-1,4-naphthaquinol-bis(disodium phosphate). *Int. J. Radiat. Biol.* **10**, 103.

HAHN, G. M. (1968). Failure of Chinese hamster cells to repair sub-lethal damage when X-irradiated in the plateau of growth. *Nature* (Lond.) **217**, 741.

HARRISON, P. R. (1968). Studies of potential radiosensitizing agents. Inhibition of nucleic acid synthesis by Synkavit (2-methyl-1,4-naphthaquinol-bis(disodium phosphate)) in Ehrlich mouse ascites tumour cells. *Brit. J. Cancer* **22**, 274.

HOLTHUSEN, H. (1921). *Pflügers Arch. f. d. ges. Physiol.* **187**, 1.

HOSHINO, T., NAGAI, M., SATO, F., SANO, K. & WATARI, T. (1970). Bromouridine (BUdR) as a radiosensitizing agent of malignant brain tumours, in *Radiation Protection and Sensitization.* Ed. H. Moroson and M. Quintiliani. Taylor and Francis, London, p. 492.

HUMPHREY, R. M., DEWEY, W. C. & CORK, A. (1963). Effect of oxygen in mammalian cells sensitized to radiation by incorporation of 5-bromodeoxyuridine into the DNA. *Nature* (Lond.) **198**, 268.

KAPLAN, H. S. (1970). Radiosensitization by the halogenated pyrimidine analogues; laboratory and clinical investigations, in *Radiation Protection and Sensitization.* Ed. H. Moroson and M. Quintiliani. Taylor and Francis, London, p. 35.

KAPLAN, H. S., ZAVARINE, R. & EARLE, J. (1962). Interaction of the oxygen effect and radiosensitization produced by base analogues incorporated into deoxyribonucleic acid. *Nature* (Lond.) **194**, 662.

KORNBERG, A. (1969). Active center of DNA polymerase. *Science* **163**, 1410.

KRISHNAMURTHI, S., SHANTA, V. & KRISHNAN NAIR, M. (1967). Studies of chemical sensitization in the radiotherapy of oral and cervical carcinomas. *Cancer* **20**, 822.

KUPFER, D. & PEETS, L. (1968). Inhibition of cortisol metabolism *in vitro* by 2-methyl-naphthoquinone (Menadione) – a possible interpretation of the potentiation of cortisol activity *in vivo*. *Experientia* **24**, 893.

LACASSAGNE, A. (1942). Chute de la sensibilité aux rayons X chez la souris nouveau-née en état d'asphyxie. *C. r. hebd. Séanc. Acad. Sci.* Paris **215**, 231.

Lerman, L. S. (1961). Structural considerations in the interaction of DNA and acridines. *J. molec. Biol.* **3,** 18.

Letnansky, K. (1968). Unterschiede der Fermentmuster verschiedener Stämme des Ehrlich-Ascitestumor. *Z. Krebsforsch.* **70,** 222.

Madoc-Jones, H. (1964). Variations in radiosensitivity of a mammalian cell line with phase of the growth cycle. *Nature* (Lond.) **203,** 983.

Marrian, D. H. (1959). Studies of potential radiosensitizing agents. An effect of tetra-sodium 2-methyl-1:4-naphthohydroquinone diphosphate (Synkavit) on the Ehrlich mouse ascites tumour. *Brit. J. Cancer* **13,** 461.

Marrian, D. H. (1965). Cit. Mitchell, J. S. (1965), p. 320.

Marrian, D. H., Marshall, B. & Mitchell, J. S. (1961). Laboratory and clinical studies of some quinol diphosphates and related compounds as chemical radiosensitizers and the development of a radioactive drug. *Chemotherapia* **3,** 225.

Marrian, D. H., Mitchell, J. S., Bull, C. H., King, E. A. & Szaz, K. F. (1969). Labelled compound related to Synkavit and its uptake in certain human tumours studied by radio-isotope scanning. *Acta radiol. Ther. Phys. Biol.* **8,** 221.

Mitchell, J. S. (1960). *Studies in Radiotherapeutics.* Harvard University Press, Cambridge, Massachusetts, and Blackwell Scientific Publications, Oxford, 274 p.; see pp. 58, 117, 147–166.

Mitchell, J. S. (1965). An attempt to develop a radioactive drug. *Clin. Radiol.* **16,** 305.

Mitchell, J. S. (1967). Strahlensensibilisierende Substanzen und ihr Einfluss auf die Strahlenempfindlichkeit von Tumouren. *Deutscher Röntgenkongress 1967.* Urban und Schwarzenberg, München, Berlin, Wien. Teil B, S.324.

Mitchell, J. S. (1968b). Applied science and the development of radiotherapy – past, present and future. The Silvanus Thompson Memorial Lecture. *Brit. J. Radiol.* **41,** 729.

Mitchell, J. S., Brinkley, D. & Haybittle, J. L. (1965). Clinical trial of radiosensitizers, including Synkavit and oxygen inhaled at atmospheric pressure. *Acta radiol. Ther. Phys. Biol.* **3,** 329.

Mitchell, J. S. & Marrian, D. H. (1965). Radiosensitization of cells by a derivative of 2-methyl-1,4-naphthoquinone, in *Biochemistry of Quinones.* Ed. R. A. Morton. Academic Press, London and New York, Chap. 15, p. 503.

Mitchell, J. S. & Simon-Reuss, I. (1947). Combination of some effects of X-radiation and a synthetic vitamin K substitute. *Nature* (Lond.) **160,** 98.

Mitchell, J. S., Simon-Reuss, I. & King, E. A. (1960). Some recent laboratory studies of chemical radiosensitizers. *Acta Unio. Int. contra Canc.* **16,** No. 5, 1201.

MOROSON, H. & QUINTILIANI, M. (1970). Radiation Protection and Sensitization. *Proc. Second Int. Symposium on Radiosensitizing and Radioprotective Drugs*. Rome. 6–8 May, 1969. Taylor and Francis, London. 524 p.

NEVILLE, D. M. & DAVIES, D. R. (1966). The interaction of acridine dyes with DNA: an X-ray diffraction and optical investigation. *J. molec. Biol.* **17**, 57.

NICOLAU, C., KÖRNER, O. & CRISTEA, A. (1966). Spin-transfer in molecular complexes of biomolecules with radiosensitizers. *Studia biophysica* (Berlin) **1**, 59.

NICOLAU, C. KÖRNER, O. & CRISTEA, A. (1967). Spin-transfer in molecular complexes of biomolecules with radiosensitizers. *Rev. roum. Phys.* **12**, 95.

OSTERBERG, K. A. & WATTENBERG, L. W. (1961). Co-enzyme Q concentration in proliferative lesions of liver. *Proc. Soc. exp. Biol. Med.* **108**, 300.

SCOTT, O. C. A. & STURROCK, J. E. (1968). Search for radiosensitization of ascites tumour cells by indanetrione. *Int. J. Radiat. Biol.* **13**, 573.

SHANTA, V., KRISHNAMURTHI, S. & SASTRI, D. V. L. N. (1969). Combined therapy in buccal mucosal cancers. *Int. Radiol. Congress*, Tokyo.

SHEHATA, A. M. EL-TABEY (1961). Effect of combined action of ionizing radiation and chemical preservatives on micro-organisms. I. Vitamin K_5 as a sensitizing agent. *Radiation Res.* **15**, 78.

SILVERMAN, G. J. (1963). In *Exploration in Future Food-processing Techniques*. Ed. S. A. Goldblith. M.I.T., Cambridge, Mass., p. 19. Cit. Bridges, B. A. (1969). *Adv. in Radiation Biology*, Academic Press, New York, Vol. 3, p. 123.

SILVERMAN, G. J., SHEHATA, A. M. EL-T. & GOLDBLITH, S. A. (1962). The radiosensitivity of *Escherichia coli* and *Streptoccocus faecalis* as influenced by Vitamin K_5 and its analogs. *Radiation Res.* **16**, 432.

SINGH, B. B., SHENOY, M. A. & GOPAL-AYENGAR, A. R. (1970). Mechanisms of radiosensitization by some sulphydryl poisons, in *Radiation, Protection and Sensitization*. Ed. H. Moroson and M. Quintiliani. Taylor and Francis, London, p. 159.

SLATER, J. P. (1966). Abstr. 3rd Meet. Fed. Europ. Biochem. Soc., Warsaw, p. 48.

SLATER, J. P. (1967). Deoxyribonucleic acid polymerase from Ehrlich ascites-tumour cells and other sources. Proc. Biochem. Soc. 22–23 June 1967. *Biochem. J.* **104**, No. 2, 30P.

SUGIMURA, T., OKABE, K. & BABA, T. (1962). Studies on ubiquinone (coenzyme Q) in neoplastic tissues. *Gann* **53**, 171.

SZYBALSKI, W. (1960). Ultraviolet light sensitivity and other biological and physico-chemical properties of halogenated DNA. *Proc. 3rd Int. Congr. Photobiology*, Copenhagen, 1960. Ed. B. Chr. Christensen and B. Buchmann. Elsevier, Amsterdam, p. 543.

TANAKA, Y. & TAKAHASHI, M. (1970). Clinical studies of intra-arterial infusion of 5-bromodeoxyuridine plus 5-fluorouracil and radiation, in *Radiation Protection and Sensitization*. Ed. H. Moroson and M. Quintiliani, Taylor and Francis, London, p. 485.

THODAY, J. M. & READ, J. (1947). Effect of oxygen on the frequency of chromosome aberrations produced by X-rays. *Nature* (Lond.) **160,** 608.

TRANZER, J. P. & PEARSE, A. G. E. (1963). Cytochemical demonstration of ubiquinones in animal tissues. *Nature* (Lond.) **199,** 1063.

VAN PUTTEN, L. M. (1968). Tumour reoxygenation during fractionated radiotherapy; studies with a transplantable mouse osteosarcoma. *Europ. J. Cancer* **4,** 173.

VAN PUTTEN. L. M. & KALLMAN, R. F. (1968). The oxygenation status of a transplantable tumour during fractionated radiation therapy. *J. Nat. Cancer Inst.* **40,** 441.

VERMUND, H. & GOLLIN, F. F. (1968). Mechanisms of action of radiotherapy and chemotherapeutic adjuvants. A review. *Cancer* **21,** 58.

WATTENBERG, L. W. (1961). Histochemical studies of the effects of coenzyme Q_{10} and menadione on oxidative enzymes in normal and neoplastic cells, in *Ciba Foundation Symposium on Quinones in Electron Transport*. Ed. G. E. W. Wolstenholme and C. M. O'Connor. J. and A. Churchill, London, p. 367.

WERNER, R. (1905). Zur chemischen Imitation der biologischen Strahlenwirkung. *Münch. med. Wschr.* **52,** 691.

WILLSON, R. L. (1970). The reaction of oxygen with radiation-induced free radicals in DNA and related compounds. *Int. J. Radiat. Biol.* **17,** 349.

ZAMENHOF, S., DE GIOVANNI, R. & GREER, S. (1958). Induced gene unstabilization. *Nature* (Lond.) **181,** 827.

ZIMBRICK, J. D., WARD, J. F. & MYERS, L. S. (1969). Studies on the chemical basis of cellular radiosensitization by 5-bromo-uracil substitution in DNA. I. Pulse- and steady-state radiolysis of 5-bromouracil and thymine. *Int. J. Radiat. Biol.* **16,** 505.

ZIMBRICK, J. D., WARD, J. F. & MYERS, L. S. (1969). Studies on the chemical basis of cellular radiosensitization by 5-bromouracil substitution in DNA. II. Pulse- and steady-state radiolysis of bromouracil substituted and unsubstituted DNA. *Int. J. Radiat. Biol.* **16,** 525.

The Possibilities of Radioactive Drugs (pp. 50–67)

ANDREWS, K. J. M., BULTITUDE, F., EVANS, E. A., GRONOW, M., LAMBERT, R. W. & MARRIAN, D. H. (1962). A radioactive drug: 2-methyl-6-tritio-1,4-naphthaquinol-bis(disodium phosphate) and 2-methyl-5,6,7,-tritritio-1,4-naphthaquinol-bis(disodium phosphate). *J. Chem. Soc.* 3440.

ARIEL, I. M. & PACK, G. T. (1960). The treatment of inoperable cancer of the biliary system with radioactive (I^{131}) rose bengal. *Amer. J. Röentgenol.* **83,** 474.

DAY, E. D., PLANINSEK, J. A. & PRESSMAN, D. (1959). Localization *in vivo* of radio-iodinated anti-rat fibrin antibodies and radio-iodinated rat fibrinogen in the Murphy rat lymphosarcoma and in other transplantable rat tumours. *J. Nat. Cancer Inst.* **22,** 413.

DENDY, P. P. (1969). Selective uptake of a radioactive drug into human tumour cells growing in tissue culture. *Acta Radiol. Ther. Phys. Biol.* **8,** 514.

GANATRA, R. D., MANI, R. S., RAMNATH, P., MEHTA, M. N., DESAI, K. B. & DESAI, C. N. (1966). A new radiopharmaceutical agent for tumour scanning. *Radiology* **87,** 750.

GANATRA, R. D., RAMANATHAN, P., PATEL, M. C., MEHTA, M. N., SHARMA, S. M., MANI, R. S., NORONHA, O. P. D. & BLAU, M. (1968). Radioiodinated Synkol as a tumor localizing agent. *J. Nuclear Med.* **9,** 318.

GANATRA, R. D., RAMANATHAN, P., PATEL, M. C., MEHTA, M. N., SHAHANI, S. N., SHARMA, S. M., MANI, R. S., NORONHA, O. P. D. & BLAU, M. (1969). Radioiodinated Synkol as a tumour-localizing agent. *Medical Radioisotope Scintigraphy.* International Atomic Agency, Vienna, Vol. II, p. 25.

GANATRA, R. D. (1969). Personal communication.

GEHAN, E. A. (1961). The determination of the number of patients required in a preliminary and a follow-up trial of a new chemotherapeutic agent. *J. Chron. Dis.* **13,** 346.

HAMILTON, J. G. (1942). Use of radioactive tracers in biology and medicine. *Radiology* **39,** 541.

HAMILTON, J. G., DURBIN, P. W., ASLING, C. W. & JOHNSTON, M. E. (1956). Physiological and biochemical studies of astatine-211 (Eka-iodine). *Proc. Int. Conf. on Peaceful Uses of Atomic Energy,* Geneva 1955. United Nations, New York. Vol. 10. Radioactive Isotopes and Nuclear Radiations in Medicine, p. 175 (P/206).

HARBERS, E. (1961). Autoradiographie, in *Kunstliche Radioaktive Isotope in Physiologie, Diagnostik und Therapie.* Hrsg. H. Schwiegk u. F. Turba, Zweite Auflage, Springer, Berlin, Göttingen, Heidelberg, 1. Bd. 321 (see p. 343).

HODGSON, A. (1968). *Studies related to the synthesis of a tritiated derivative of 2-methyl-1,4-naphthoquinone.* Ph.D. Dissertation, University of Cambridge.

HORWITZ, H., GREGG, D. McC., MARRIAN, D. H., MARSHALL, B. & MITCHELL, J. S. (1959). Clinical and laboratory studies of the therapeutic possibilities of tritiated Synkavit, mainly by intra-arterial administration. *Acta Rad.* (Stockh.). Suppl. 188, p. 111.

REFERENCES

KESTON, A. S., BALL, R. P., FRANTZ, V. K. & PALMER, W. W. (1942). Storage of radioactive iodine in a metastasis from thyroid carcinoma. *Science* **95**, 362.

KOTTMANN, K. (1935). Experimentelle Untersuchungen mit substituierten Naphtalinsulfosäuren im Hinblick auf Blutgerinnung, Blutfärbung und Tumoraffinität. *Schweiz. med. Wschr.* **16**, 533.

KROLL, K. H., STRAUSS, S. F. & NECHELES, H. (1941). Studies on the detection of abscesses and tumours. III. Concentration and detection of a radioactive substance in abscesses. *J. Lab. Clin. Med.* **27**, 50.

LETTRÉ, H. (1946). Ergebnisse und Probleme der Mitosegiftforschung. *Naturwissenschaften* **33**, 75.

MARRIAN, D. H. (1957). Tritium-labelled 2-methyl-1:4-naphthaquinone and confirmation of the structure of its adduct with sodium hydrogen sulphite. *J. Chem. Soc.*, p. 499.

MARRIAN, D. H. & MAXWELL, D. R. (1956a). Tracer studies of potential radiosensitizing agents. Tetrasodium 2-^{14}C-methyl-1:4-naphthohydroquinone diphosphate. *Brit. J. Cancer* **10**, 575.

MARRIAN, D. H. & MAXWELL, D. R. (1956b). Tracer studies of potential radiosensitizing agents. Tetrasodium 2-methyl-3-^{82}bromo-1:4-naphthohydroquinone diphosphate and tetrasodium 2:3-dimethyl-5:6-di-^{131}I-iodo-1:4-benzohydroquinone diphosphate. *Brit. J. Cancer* **10**, 739.

MARRIAN, D. H., MITCHELL, J. S., BULL, C. H., KING, E. A. & SZAZ, K. F. (1969). Labelled compound related to Synkavit and its uptake in certain human tumours studied by radio-isotope scanning. *Acta Radiol. Ther. Phys. Biol.* **8**, 221.

MAXWELL, D. R. (1954). Some experiments with labelled compounds related to 2-methyl-1:4-naphthohydroquinone diphosphate (Synkavit). *2nd Radio-isotope Conference*. Oxford. Butterworths, London, p. 200.

MAXWELL, D. R. (1955). *Studies of chemotherapeutic agents, which incorporate radioactive atoms and may concentrate in malignant tumour cells*. Ph.D. Dissertation, University of Cambridge.

MITCHELL, J. S. (1949). *Ann. Rep. Brit. Emp. Cancer Campaign* **27**, 214.

MITCHELL, J. S. (1953). Laboratory studies and clinical therapeutic trials of some chemical radiosensitizers. *Acta Radiol.* (Stockh.) Suppl. **116**, 431.

MITCHELL, J. S. (1955). *Laboratory studies and clinical trials of some chemical radiosensitizers. Radiobiology Symposium*, Liège, 1954. Butterworths, London, p. 170. See also Addendum, p. 182.

MITCHELL, J. S. (1962). Über die Möglichkeit der Verwendung strahlensensibilisierender Substanzen. In *Strahlenschutz in Forschung und Praxis*. Ed. H.-J. Melching, H. R. Beck, H.-A. Ladner und E. Scherer. Rombach, Freiburg i. Br., Band 2, S.139.

MITCHELL, J. S. (1963). An attempt to develop a radioactive drug for cancer therapy. *Proc. Roy. Soc. Med.* **56**, 651.

MITCHELL, J. S. (1964). Zur Entwicklung radioaktiver Pharmaka. *Deutsch-Englische Medizinische Rundschau* **2,** 524.

MITCHELL, J. S. (1965a). An attempt to develop a radioactive drug. *Clinical Radiology* **16,** 305. The Robert Knox Memorial Lecture, 1965.

MITCHELL, J. S. (1965b). Über die Möglichkeit der Verwendung radioaktiver Pharmaka. *Strahlentherapie* **127,** 497.

MITCHELL, J. S. (1965c). A review of clinical and laboratory studies of radiosensitisers in radiotherapy. Paper given at 1st International Symposium on Radiosensitisers and Radioprotectors, Milan, 1964. *Progr. Biochem. Pharmacol.* **1,** 335. Karger, Basel, New York.

MITCHELL, J. S. (1966). Ein Beitrag zur Untersuchung radioaktiver Pharmaka. *Strahlentherapie* **131,** 331.

MITCHELL, J. S. (1967a). The use of tritium-labelled compounds. Chapter from *Modern Trends in Radiotherapy*. Ed. T. J. Deeley and C. A. P. Wood. Butterworths, London. p. 187.

MITCHELL, J. S. (1967b). Strahlensensibilisierende Substanzen und ihr Einfluss auf die Strahlenempfindlichkeit von Tumoren, *Deutscher Röntgenkongress 1967*, Urban und Schwarzenberg, München, Berlin, Wien, Teil B. Strahlenbehandlung und Strahlenbiologie, S.324.

MITCHELL, J. S. (1969). Diagnostische und therapeutische Anwendungen der radioaktiven Pharmaka in der Tumorbehandlung. (Radioactive drugs in the treatment ond diagnosis of tumours). *Kerntechnik* **II,** No. 6, 346.

MITCHELL, J. S. (1970). Über die Möglichkeit der Entwicklung radioaktiver Pharmaka. Festvortrag. *Vereinigung deutscher Strahlenschutz-Ärzte.* 10. Tagung, Würzburg, 24.10.69. Thieme, Stuttgart. (In press.)

MITCHELL, J. S., KING, E. A., MARRIAN, D. H. & CHIPPERFIELD, B. (1963). Investigation of a radioactive drug (TRA 119) with special reference to autoradiographic and related studies. *Acta radiol. Ther. Phys. Biol.* **1,** 321.

MOORE, G. E. (1948). Radioactive localization of brain tumours. *J. Amer. Med. Ass.* **137,** 1228.

PHILLIPS, A. F. (1954). The gamma-ray dose in carcinoma of the thyroid treated by radio-iodine. *Acta radiol.* (Stockh.) **41,** 533.

PHILLIPS, A. F. (1955). *Autoradiographic studies in connection with the clinical use of radioactive isotopes.* M.D. Thesis, University of Edinburgh.

PHILLIPS, A. F. (1957). The choice of a radioactive isotope for treatment of carcinoma of the thyroid. *Brit. J. Radiol.* **30,** 247.

PHILLIPS, A. F., HAYBITTLE, J. L. & NEWBERY, G. R. (1960). Use of Iodine-124 for the treatment of carcinoma of the thyroid. *Acta Un. int. contr. Canc.* **16,** 1434.

POCHIN, E. E. (1969). Personal communication.

RAJEWSKY, M. F. (1965). Thymidin-Inkorporation und O_2-Konzentration in Explantaten normaler und maligner Gewebe "in vitro". *Naturwissenschaften* **52**, 341.

SEIDLIN, S. M., ROSSMAN, J., OSHRY, E. & SIEGEL, E. (1949). Radioiodine therapy of metastases from carcinoma of the thyroid. (A six year progress report). *J. clin. Endocrin.* **9**, 1122.

SHOOP, J. D. (1969). Functional hepatoma demonstrated with rose bengal scanning. *Amer. J. Röentgenol.* **107**, 51.

SILVER, I. A., CATER, D. B., MARRIAN, D. H. & MARSHALL, B. (1962). Tritiated tetra-sodium 2-methyl-1:4-naphthaquinol diphosphate for treatment of spontaneous tumours in animals. *Acta radiol.* (Stockh.) **58**, 281.

SIMON-REUSS, I. (1961). H^3 incorporation into ascites tumour and tissue culture cells exposed to Synkavit and its tritiated analogue. *Acta radiol.* (Stockh.) **56**, 49.

SPAR, I. L., BALE, W. F., MARRACK, D., DEWEY, W. C., MCCARDLE, R. J. & HARPER, P. V. (1967). ^{131}I-labelled antibodies to human fibrinogen. Diagnostic studies and therapeutic trials. *Cancer* **20**, 865.

THOMAS, E. W. (1970). Personal communication.

WASSERMANN, A. v., KEYSSER, F. & WASSERMANN, M. (1911). Beiträge zum Problem: Geschwülste von der Blutbahn aus therapeutisch zu beeinflussen. (Auf Grund chemotherapeutischer Versuche an tumorkranken Tieren). *Dtsch. med. Wschr.* **37**, 2389.

Problems involved in the practical dosage of the tritiated drugs (pp. 67–74)

BLEECKEN, S. (1964). Tritium-Mikrodosimetrie. *Strahlentherapie* **125**, 145.

CHIPPERFIELD, B. (1967a). Tritium uptake, half-lives and radiation doses in tissues of cancer patients treated with tritiated 2-methyl-1:4-naphthaquinol diphosphate. *Int. J. Cancer* **2**, 381.

CHIPPERFIELD, B. (1967b). Excretion of tritium after therapeutic injections of tritiated 2-methyl-1:4-naphthaquinol diphosphate in cancer patients. *Int. J. Cancer* **2**, 396.

CLEAVER, J. E. (1967). *Thymidine metabolism and cell kinetics.* North-Holland Publ. Co., Amsterdam.

GOODHEART, C. R. (1961). Radiation dose calculation in cells containing intranuclear tritium. *Radiation Res.* **15**, 767.

HALL, E. J., OLIVER, R. & BEDFORD, J. S. (1967). The relative biological effectiveness of tritium beta-particles compared to gamma-radiation – its dependence on dose-rate. *Brit. J. Radiol.* **40**, 704.

KÜNKEL, H. A. (1962). Zur Frage der Strahlenbelastung des Zellkerns durch Inkorporation von tritium-markiertem Thymidin. *Strahlentherapie* **118**, 46.

MITCHELL, J. S. (1966). Ein Beitrag zur Untersuchung radioaktiver Pharmaka. *Strahlentherapie* **131**, 331; see pp. 338–340.

MITCHELL, J. S. (1968). Applied science and the development of radiotherapy – past, present and future. *Brit. J. Radiol.* **41**, 729; see pp. 742–744.

RITZL, F. (1968). Der Umbau des Menadion-Diphosphat-Tetranatriumsalzes (Synkavit) im Menschen, in *Radioisotope in Pharmakokinetik und klinische Biochemie. 6. Jahrestagung der Gesellschaft für Nuclearmedizin E.V. 26–28. September 1968.* Wiesbaden, Buchler und Co., Braunschweig, Frankfurt. Vortrag Nr. 79.

STEWART, F. S. (1964). The calculation of radiation dose from distributed sources of tritium. *Int. J. Radiat. Biol.* **8,** 545.

STRAUSS, B. S. (1958). The genetic effect of incorporated radioisotopes: the transmutation problem. *Radiation Res.* **8,** 234.

TÄGDER, K. & SCHEUERMANN, W. (1970). Estimation of absorbed doses in the cell nucleus after incorporation of ^{3}H- or ^{14}C-labeled Thymidine. *Radiation Res.* **41,** 202.

Some considerations of the mechanisms of the therapeutic actions of ionizing radiations (pp. 74–86)

ALEXANDER, P. (1967). Personal communication.

ALEXANDER, P., DEAN, C. J., LEHMANN, A. R., ORMEROD, M. G., FELDSCHREIBER, P. & SERIANNI, R. W. (1970). The repair of DNA and the mode of action of sensitizers and protectors in biological systems of different complexity, in *Radiation Protection and Sensitization,* Ed. H. Moroson and M. Quintiliani. Taylor and Francis, London, p. 15.

ALPER, T. (1961). Variability in the oxygen effect observed with microorganisms. Part II. Escherichia coli B. *Int. J. Radiat. Biol.* **3,** 369.

ALPER, T. (1963). Lethal mutations and cell death. Eighth Douglas Lea Memorial Lecture. *Phys. Med. Biol.* **8,** 365.

ALPER, T. (1968). Low oxygen enhancement ratios for radiosensitive bacterial strains, and the probable interaction of two types of primary lesion. *Nature* (Lond.) **217,** 862.

ALPER, T. (1968). Radiation-induced lethality and DNA strand breakage: the relevance of the oxygen effect. *Int. J. Radiat. Biol.* **14,** 83.

AOKI, S., BOYCE, R. P. & HOWARD-FLANDERS, P. (1966). Sensitization of *Escherichia coli* to radiation by bromouracil: excessive post-irradiation breakdown of deoxyribonucleic acid without concomitant synthesis. *Nature* (Lond.) **209,** 686.

ATWOOD, K. C. & NORMAN, A. (1949). On the interpretation of multi-hit survival curves. *Proc. nat. Acad. Sci.* (Wash.) **35,** 696.

BACQ, Z. M. & ALEXANDER, P. (1961). *Fundamentals of Radiobiology.* 2nd Ed., Pergamon Press, Oxford, London, New York, Paris. 555 p.

BALAZS, E. A., DAVIES, J. V., PHILLIPS, G. O. & YOUNG, M. D. (1967). Transient intermediates in the radiolysis of hyaluronic acid. *Radiation Res.* **31,** 243.

REFERENCES

BAUER, R. D., JOHANSEN, R. & THOMASSON, W. A. (1969). Alterations of DNA-histone interactions following irradiation. *Int. J. Radiat. Biol.* **16,** 575.

BRINKMAN, R. & LAMBERTS, H. B. (1958). Direct registration of an instantaneous X-ray effect in rats and man. *Nature* (Lond.) **181,** 774.

BRINKMAN, R. & LAMBERTS, H. B. (1960). Examples of immediate low-level X-ray effects; their significance for the study of chemical protection in *Immediate and Low Level Effects of Ionizing Radiation,* Ed. A. A. Buzzati-Traverso, Taylor and Francis, London, p. 167.

BRINKMAN, R. & LAMBERTS, H. B. (1966). Radiopathology of extracellular structures, in *Current Topics in Radiation Research,* Ed. E. M. Ebert and A. Howard. North-Holland Publ. Co., Amsterdam, Vol. II, Chap. VI. p. 279.

BRUCE, A. K. & MALCHMAN, W. H. (1965). Radiation sensitization of *Micrococcus radiodurans, Sarcina lutea* and *Escherichia coli* by p-hydroxymercuribenzoate. *Radiation Res.* **24,** 473.

CASPERSSON, T., KLEIN, E. & RINGERTZ, N. R. (1958). Cytochemical studies of some effects of X-radiation on three ascites tumours. *Cancer Research,* **18,** 857.

CAIRNS, J. (1966). Autoradiography of HeLa Cell DNA. *J. Mol. Biol.* **15,** 372.

CRAMP, W. A. (1970). Modification of post-irradiation DNA degradation in *E. coli B/r., Radiation Protection and Sensitization,* Ed. H. Moroson and M. Quintiliani, Taylor and Francis, London, p. 155 .

EPSTEIN, S. M., BENEDETTI, E. L., SHINAZUKA, H., BARTUS, B. & FARBER, E. (1970). Altered and distorted DNA from a premalignant liver lesion induced by 2-fluorenylacetamide. *Chem.-Biol. Interactions* **1,** 113.

ERNST, H. (1961). Strahlenbedingte Frühveränderungen an Zell-kern-Proteinen. I. Histone und nukleare Globuline von Thymus und Milz. *Z. Naturforsch,* **16b,** 329.

ERNST, H. (1963). Zur Frage der Dosis-Abhängigkeit der strahlenin-duzierten Nukleoprotein-Verminderung im Zellkern von Leber, Milz und Thymus. *Naturwissenschaften* **50,** 333.

EULER, H. v. & HEVESY, G. v. (1942). Wirkung der Röntgenstrahlen auf den Umsatz der Nukleinsäure im Jensen-Sarkom. *Det. Kgl. Danske Videnskabernes Selskab. Biol. Medd.* **17,** No. 8.

EULER, H. v. & HEVESY, G. v. (1944). Wirkung der Röntgenstrahlen auf den Umsatz der Nukleinsäure im Jensen-Sarkom. II. *Arkiv. för kemi, mineralogi o. geologi.* **17A,** No. 30.

FOX, M. (1968). The effect of halogenated nucleosides on the sensitivity of a mouse lymphoma P388F to X-rays and methyl methanesulphon-ate. *Int. J. Cancer* **3,** 382.

FOX, M. & LAJTHA, L. G. (1967). Continuous irradiation of P388F lymphoma *in vitro*, sensitisation by 5′-iodo-2′-deoxyuridine. *Int. J. Radiat. Biol.* **12**, 251.

FREIFELDER, D. (1968). Physico-chemical studies on X-ray inactivation of bacteriophage. *Virology* **36**, 613.

GRAY, L. H. (1959). Cellular radiobiology. *Radiation Res.* Suppl. 1, p. 73.

HAGEN, U. (1960). Labilization of deoxyribonucleic acid in thymus nucleoprotein after whole-body irradiation. *Nature* (Lond.) **187**, 1123.

HAGEN, U. (1961). Untersuchungen über die Entstehung der Thymusatrophie nach Röntenbestrahlung. II. Das Schicksal der Desoxyribonukleinsäure. *Strahlentherapie* **116**, 385.

HARBERS, E. & BACKMANN, R. (1956). Untersuchungen über den Einfluss von Röntgenstrahlen auf die Desoxyribonukleinsäure im Walker-Carcinom der Ratte. *Exp. Cell Res.* **10**, 125.

HEWITT, H. B. (1963). Effects on organized systems in the light of cellular radiobiology, in *Radiation effects in physics, chemistry and biology.* Proc. Sec. Int. Congr. Radiation Res., Harrogate, 1962. Ed. M. Ebert and A. Howard. North-Holland Publ. Co., Amsterdam, p. 234; see p. 236.

HIDVÉGI, E. J., BÖLÖNI, E., HOLLAND, J., ANTONI, F. & VÁRTERÉSZ, V. (1970). The effect of whole-body X-irradiation of guinea pigs on liver ribonucleic acid synthesis. *Biochem. J.* **116**, 503.

HUG, O. u. Kellerer, A. M. (1966). *Stochastik der Strahlenwirkung.* Springer, Berlin, Heidelberg, New York, 137 p; see p. 43.

HUMPHREY, R. M. & SINCLAIR, W. K. (1963). The relative biological effectiveness of 22-MeVp X-rays, Cobalt-60 gamma rays, and 200 Kv X-rays. VIII. *Radiation Res.* **20**, 593.

HUTCHINSON, F. (1966). The molecular basis for radiation effects on cells. *Cancer Res.* **26**, 2045.

KAPLAN, H. S. (1970). Radiosensitization by the halogenated pyrimidine analogues: laboratory and clinical investigations, in *Radiation Protection and Sensitization.* Ed. H. Moroson and M. Quintiliani. Taylor and Francis, London, p. 35.

KILLANDER, D., RICHARDS, B. M. & RINGERTZ, N. R. (1962). The effect of X-radiation on nuclear nucleotide content as studied by ultra-violet-microspectrophotometry on tumour cells. *Exp. Cell Res.* **27**, 321.

LAMPERT, F. (1969). Feinstruktur und Trockengewicht menschlicher Chromosomen. *Naturwissenschaften* **56**, 629.

LETT, J. T. & ALEXANDER, P. (1966). *Ann. Rep. Brit. Emp. Cancer Camp.* 35.

LETT, J. T., CALDWELL, I., DEAN, C. J. & ALEXANDER, P. (1967). Rejoining of X-ray induced breaks in the DNA of leukaemia cells. *Nature* (Lond.) **214**, 790.

REFERENCES

LETT, J. T., CALDWELL, I. & LITTLE, J. G. (1970). Repair of X-ray damage to the DNA in *Micrococcus radiodurans:* the effect of 5-bromodeoxyuridine. *J. Mol. Biol.* **48,** 395.

LETT, J. T., FELDSCHREIBER, P., LITTLE, J. G., STEELE, K. & DEAN, C. J. (1967). The repair of X-ray damage to the deoxyribonucleic acid in *Micrococcus radiodurans:* a study of the excision process. *Proc. Roy. Soc. B.* **167,** 184.

LETT, J. T., PARKINS, G., ALEXANDER, P. & ORMEROD, M. G. (1964). Mechanisms of sensitization to X-rays of mammalian cells by 5-bromodeoxyuridine. *Nature* (Lond.) **203,** 593.

LUND, E. & ROSENGREN, B. (1966). Survival of HeLa cells after large doses of X-radiation. *Int. J. Radiat. Biol.* **11,** 99.

McGRATH, R. A. & WILLIAMS, R. W. (1966). Reconstruction *in vivo* of irradiated *Escherichia coli* deoxyribonucleic acid; the rejoining of broken peices. *Nature* (Lond.) **212,** 534.

McGRATH, R. A., WILLIAMS, R. W. & SWARTZENDRUBER, D. C. (1966). Breakdown of DNA in X-irradiated *Escherichia coli. Biophysical J.* **6,** 113.

MITCHELL, J. S. (1940). Increase in ultra-violet absorption of cytoplasm after therapeutic X- and gamma-irradiation. *Nature* (Lond.) **146,** 272.

MITCHELL, J. S. (1942a). Disturbance of nucleic acid metabolism produced by therapeutic doses of X- and gamma-radiations. Part 1. Methods of investigation. *Brit. J. Exp. Path.* **23,** 285.

MITCHELL, J. S. (1942b). Disturbance of nucleic acid metabolism produced by therapeutic doses of X- and gamma-radiations. Part 2. Accumulation of pentose nucleotides in cytoplasm after irradiation. *Brit. J. Exp. Path.* **23,** 296.

MITCHELL, J. S. (1942c). Disturbance of nucleic acid metabolism produced by therapeutic doses of X- and gamma-radiations. Part 3. Inhibition of synthesis of thymonucleic acid by radiation. *Brit. J. Exp. Path.* **23,** 309.

MITCHELL, J. S. (1943). Metabolic effects of therapeutic doses of X- and gamma-radiations. *Brit. J. Radiol.* **16,** 339.

MITCHELL, J. S. (1944). Disturbance of nucleic acid metabolism produced by therapeutic doses of X- and gamma-radiations. *Brit. Emp. Can. Camp. 21st Annual Report*, p. 62.

MITCHELL, J. S. (1956). Some problems of radiotherapeutics. *Proc. Int. Conf. on Peaceful Uses of Atomic Energy*, Geneva, 1955, United Nations, New York, Vol. 10, Radioactive Isotopes and Nuclear Radiations in Medicine, p. 25; see pp. 37, 38 (P/446).

MITCHELL, J. S. (1956). The 'macromolecular lesion' involving deoxyribonucleic acid in radiobiology and radiotherapy. *J. Colloid Science* **11,** 317.

MITCHELL, J. S. (1960). *Studies in Radiotherapeutics.* Blackwell Scientific Publications, Oxford and Harvard University Press, Cambridge, Massachusetts, see p. 26 and pp. 48–59.

MITCHELL, J. S. (1966). Some aspects of the effects of radiations on the metabolism of tissues and tumours. Chapter in *Encyclopaedia of Medical Radiology*, Vol. II, Part I. Ed. A. Zuppinger. Springer, Berlin, Heidelberg, New York, pp. 355–486; see pp. 448–449.

MITCHELL, J. S. (1968a). Applications of radiation chemistry in radiobiology and radiotherapeutics, in *Radiation chemistry of aqueous systems*. Proc. 19th L. Farkas Memorial Symposium, Jerusalem, 27–29 Dec. 1967. Ed. Gabriel Stein. The Weizmann Science Press of Israel, Jerusalem. Interscience Publishers, John Wiley, London, New York, Sydney, p. 287.

MITCHELL, J. S. (1968b). Applied science and the development of radiotherapy – past, present and future. The Silvanus Thompson Memorial Lecture, *Brit. J. Radiol.* **41,** 729; see pp. 733–735.

MITCHELL, J. S. (1968). Some recent studies in radiotherapeutics. *J. Obstet. Gynaec. Brit. Cmwlth.* **75,** 1268.

MOSELEY, B. E. B. & LASER, H. (1965). Repair of X-ray damage in Micrococcus radiodurans. *Proc. Roy. Soc. B.* **162,** 210.

MUNSON, R. J., NEARY, G. J., BRIDGES, B. A. & PRESTON, R. J. (1967). The sensitivity of *Escherichia coli* to ionizing particles of different LETs. *Int. J. Radiat. Biol.* **13,** 205.

MUNSON, R. J., NEARY, G. J., BRIDGES, B. A. & PRESTON, R. J. (1968). Radiation sensitivity of *E. coli* and LET. *Int. J. Radiat. Biol.* **14,** 85.

NIAS. A. H. W., GILBERT, C. W., LAJTHA, L. G. & LANGE, C. S. (1965). Clone-size analysis in the study of cell growth following single or during continuous irradiation. *Int. J. Radiat. Biol.* **9,** 275.

POLLARD, E. C. & WELLER, P. K. (1968). Post-irradiation permeability of *Escherichia coli* cells. *Radiation Res.* **35,** 722.

PUCK, T. T. & MARCUS, P. I. (1956). Action of X-rays on single mammalian cells. *J. Exp. Med.* **103,** 653.

PUCK, T. T., MARCUS, P. I. & CIECIURA, S. J. (1956). Clonal growth of mammalian cells *in vitro*. II. *J. Exp. Med.* **103,** 273; see Puck and Marcus, 1956.

RÉVÉSZ, L. & LITTBRAND, L. (1966). Proc. Int. Congr. Radiol. 1965. (Excerpta Med. Int. Congr. Series No. 105), p. 1476.

RÉVÉSZ, L. and LITTBRAND, L. (1967). *Proc. Int. Conf. Radiation Biol. and Cancer*, Kyoto, 1966. (Publ. Radiation Soc. of Japan), p. 67.

SEED, J. (1960a). Inhibition of nucleic acid synthesis caused by X-irradiation of the nucleolus. *Proc. Roy. Soc. B.* **152,** 387.

SEED, J. (1960b). X-irradiation of the nucleolus and its effect on nucleic acid synthesis, in *The Cell Nucleus* (J. S. Mitchell). Butterworths, London, pp. 49–52; see also p. 53.

SEED. J. (1966a). The synthesis of DNA, RNA and nuclear protein in normal and tumour strain cells. I. Fresh embryo human cells. *J. Cell Biol.* **28,** 233.

SEED, J. (1966b). The synthesis of DNA, RNA and nuclear protein in normal and tumour strain cells. II. Fresh embryo mouse cells. *J. Cell Biol.* **28**, 249.

SEED, J. (1966c). The synthesis of DNA, RNA and nuclear protein in normal and tumour strain cells. III. Mouse ascites tumour cells. *J. Cell Biol.* **28**, 257.

SEED, J. (1966d). The synthesis of DNA, RNA and nuclear protein in normal and tumour strain cells. IV. HeLa tumour strain cells. *J. Cell Biol.* **28**, 263.

STRAZHEVSKAYA, N. B. & STRUCHKOV, V. A. (1962) On the role of DNA supramolecular structure in cell radiation injury. *Radiobiology*, Translation of Vol. 2. AEC-tr-5428, 10.

STRAZHEVSKAYA, N. B. & STRUCHKOV, V. A. (1963). Molecular structure of DNA and radiation damage to cells in *Radiation effects in physics, chemistry and biology*. Proc. Sec. Int. Congr. Radiation Research, Harrogate, 1962. Ed. M. Ebert and A. Howard. North-Holland Publ. Co., Amsterdam, pp. 101–103 and 113.

STREFFER, C. (1969). *Strahlen-Biochemie*. Springer, Berlin, Heidelberg, New York. (Heidelberger Taschenbücher 59/60), (1965).

SWINGLE, K. F. & COLE, L. J. (1968). Early effects of ionizing radiations on nucleic acids, in *Current Topics in Radiation Research*. Ed. M. Ebert and A. Howard, North-Holland Publ. Co., Amsterdam, Vol. IV, p. 191.

TERASIMA, T. & TSUBOI, A. (1969). Mammalian cell DNA isolated with minimal shearing: a sensitive system for detecting strand breaks by radiation. *Biochim. Biophys. Acta* **174**, 309.

VAN DER SCHANS, G. P. & BLOK, J. (1970). The influence of oxygen and sulphhydryl compounds on the production of breaks in bacteriophage DNA by gamma-rays. *Int. J. Radiat. Biol.* **17**, 25.

WEBB, S. J. & BATHER, R. (1970). Infra red studies of isolated normal and tumour DNA. *Phys. Med. Biol.* **15**, 271.

WEINERT, H. & HAGEN, U. (1968). Über die Strahlenempfindlichkeit der Desoxyribonukleinsäure im Chromatin. *Strahlentherapie* **136**, 204.

WHITMORE, G. F. & TILL, J. E. (1964). Quantitation of cellular radiobiological responses. *Ann. Rev. Nuclear Science* **14**, 347.

VI. IF CURABLE, WHY NOT CURED?

A partial answer to the question and some problems of organisation (pp. 87–93)

BYATT, I. C. R. & COHEN, A. V. (1969). An attempt to quantify the economic benefits of scientific research. *Science Policy Studies*. No. 4. Department of Education and Science. H.M.S.O., London. 25 p.

Forssell, Gösta (1935). Strahlentherapie maligner Tumoren in Schweden. *Wien. klin. Wschr.* **38,** 1.

Forssell, Gösta (1930). Les lignes fondamentales de l'organisation de la lutte contre le cancer. *Ligue Nat. Belge contre le Cancer.* Bruxelles, 29 p.

More, Sir Thomas (1516). *Utopia*, Louvain. Yale Edition. Ed. E. Surtz. Yale University Press, New Haven and London, p. 78.

Papanicolaou, G. N. (1928). *Proc. 3rd Race Betterment Conf.* p. 528 (cit. McLaren, 1963).

Papanicolaou, G. N. & Traut, H. F. (1943). *Diagnosis of uterine cancer.* The New York Commonwealth Fund.

Schinz, H. R. & Zuppinger, A. (1937). *Siebzehn Jahre Strahlentherapie der Krebse: Zürcher Erfahrungen 1919–1935.* Georg Thieme, Leipzig, see pp. 17, 20.

Stockhard, C. R. & Papanicolaou, G. N. (1917). The existence of the typical oestrous cycle in the guinea pig with a study of its histology and physiological stages. *Amer. J. Anat.* **22,** 225.

World Health Organization (1966) Cancer Treatment: *Report of WHO Expert Committee,* W.H.O. Technical Report Series No. 322, W.H.O., Geneva, see p. 39.

APPENDIX

The following additional references may be of interest:

Burkitt, D. (1967). Long-term remissions following one and two-dose chemotherapy for African lymphoma. *Cancer* 20, i, 756.

Lewis, M. G., Ikonopisov, R. L., Nairn, R. C., Phillips, T. M., Hamilton Fairley, G., Bodenham, D. C. & Alexander, P. (1969). Tumour-specific antibodies in human malignant melanoma and their relationship to the extent of the disease. *Brit. med. J.* 547.

Mathé, G. (1969). Approaches to the immunological treatment of cancer in man. *Brit. med. J.* 7.

Tanneberger, S. & Bacigalupo, G. (1970). Einige Erfahrungen mit der individuellen zytostatischen Behandlung maligner Tumoren nach prätherapeutischer Zytostatika-Sensibilitätsprüfung in vitro (Onkobiogramm). *Arch. Geschwulstforsch.* **31/1,** 44.

Thomson G. P. (1969). An appeal to doctors. *Lancet*, p. 1353.

SUBJECT INDEX

AUTHOR INDEX